WHY YOU SHOULD READ THIS BOOK

Like most of us today, you probably have to carve out time in your busy schedule in order to read a book. Therefore, you don't want your time to be wasted, and you want what you read to have value for you. If you are thinking of reading this book you are most likely interested in finding answers for how you can improve your health and the health of your loved ones. I wrote this book to help you do so.

Over the course of many years as both a writer of health books and an explorer of effective self-care measures that we can all use to improve our health, I have discovered that many of the most effective solutions are to be found in nature. Such natural solutions not only offer important health benefits, they are also inexpensive, readily available, and can be as effective as any prescription or over-the-counter medication. And, as an added advantage, they are also free of the unpleasant, even dangerous, side effects so commonly caused by pharmaceutical drugs today. As this book makes clear, that is certainly the case for coconut and its oil and milk.

If you read this book to its end and, most importantly, if you apply the suggestions for improving your health that it offers on a consistent basis, I promise you that your time will not be wasted and that there is a very good chance that you will find beneficial answers to your health concerns that will make a positive difference in your life.

Thank you for choosing to read it.

OTHER WORKS BY LARRY TRIVIERI, JR.

From Square One Publishers

Apple Cider Vinegar: Nature's Most Powerful and Versatile Remedy

*The Acid-Alkaline Lifestyle: The Complete Program
for Better Health And Vitality* (with Neil Raff, MD)

The Acid-Alkaline Food Guide (with Susan Brown, PhD)

Juice Alive: The Ultimate Guide to Juicing Remedies (with Steven Bailey, ND)

Other Select Titles

Alternative Medicine: The Definitive Guide, 1st and 2nd editions (editor and
co-author with Burton Goldberg)

The American Holistic Medical Association Guide to Holistic Health

Chronic Fatigue, Fibromyalgia and Lyme Disease (with Burton Goldberg)

Novels

The Monster and Freddie Fype

Krystle's Quest

Tommy's Big Question

COCONUTS
FOR YOUR HEALTH

Nature's Most Delicious
& Effective Remedy

Larry Trivieri, Jr.

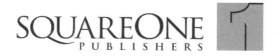

SQUAREONE
PUBLISHERS

The information and advice contained in this book are based upon the research and the personal and professional experiences of the author. They are not intended as a substitute for consulting with a health care professional. The publisher and author are not responsible for any adverse effects or consequences resulting from the use of any of the suggestions, preparations, or procedures discussed in this book. All matters pertaining to your physical health should be supervised by a health care professional. It is a sign of wisdom, not cowardice, to seek a second or third opinion.

EDITOR: Erica Shur
COVER DESIGNER: Jeannie Tudor
TYPESETTER: Gary A. Rosenberg

Square One Publishers

115 Herricks Road
Garden City Park, NY 11040
(516) 535-2010 • (877) 900-BOOK
www.squareonepublishers.com

Library of Congress Cataloging-in-Publication Data

Names: Trivieri, Larry, 1956- author.
Title: Coconuts for your health : nature's most delicious & effective remedy
/ by Larry Trivieri, Jr.
Description: Garden City Park, NY : Square One Publishers, [2018] | Includes
bibliographical references and index.
Identifiers: LCCN 2017050461 (print) | LCCN 2017053530 (ebook) | ISBN
9780757054518 | ISBN 9780757004513
Subjects: LCSH: Coconut—Health aspects. | Coconut—Nutrition. |
Coconut—Therapeutic use.
Classification: LCC QP144.C63 (ebook) | LCC QP144.C63 T75 2018 (print) | DDC
615.8/54—dc23
LC record available at https://lccn.loc.gov/2017050461

Printed in the United States of America

10   9   8   7   6   5   4   3   2   1

Contents

For my Mom,
for Everything!

Introduction

Throughout history and in cultures all around the world, the healing properties of foods and herbs have been widely recognized as one of nature's most important gifts to humankind. Two thousand five hundred years ago, Hippocrates, the renowned Father of Western Medicine for whom the Hippocratic Oath was named wrote, "Let food be thy medicine, and medicine thy food." This sage advice was followed by healers and physicians for centuries before being supplanted by the advent of modern science and medicine's shift towards drug-based therapies.

Today, few conventionally trained physicians know much, if anything, about the healing properties of foods. This fact may seem surprising, yet the reality is that the average amount of time that physicians spend learning about diet and nutrition during their eight or more years of medical school is only twenty-five hours over that entire time period. You can learn more about the importance of diet and nutrition simply by reading one or more books on the subject, including some of my own titles.

The irony of conventional medicine's reliance on drug-based medicine is that the word *drug* itself is derived from the Dutch word *drogge,* which means "to dry," as traditional healers often dried plants in order to prepare them for medicinal use. Also ironic is the fact that approximately 25 percent of all pharmaceutical drugs used by physicians today are derived from plant foods and herbs. One very common example of this is aspirin, which is derived from the herb white willow bark. Other examples include the heart medication digitalis, which is derived from the foxglove plant, and the gout drug colchicine, which comes from the autumn crocus plant. Also noteworthy is a study conducted by the World Health Organization that found that 74 percent of 119 pharmaceutical drugs derived from plants directly correlated with the ways the plants themselves are used medicinally in their native cultures.

There is a big difference between how plant foods and herbs are used to heal compared to pharmaceutical drugs used for the same purposes. By and large, researchers at drug companies seek to isolate and then synthesize what they regard to be the primary active ingredient in plant foods and herbs in order to develop their drugs. In doing so, very often the various other ingredients found in plant foods and herbs are ignored or discarded, *even though these other ingredients also play important roles in the plant foods' ability to promote healing.*

In nature, the active ingredients found in healing plants and herbs are supported and made more effective by a variety of other co-factor nutrients that work together synergistically with the active ingredient. Isolated active ingredients, acting alone, cannot always provide the same degree of health enhancing benefits without the co-factor nutrients to assist them. And when these active ingredients are synthesized to produce drugs, they no longer work in the body the same way that natural substances, from foods, do. This fact in large part explains why almost all pharmaceutical drugs, including plain aspirin (unlike the willow bark from which it is derived), carry the risk of serious, sometimes even fatal side effects. (According to both the American Medical Association and the prestigious *New England Journal of Medicine,* each year in the United States, more than 100,000 people die as a result of using properly prescribed pharmaceutical drugs taken according to their doctors' directions, and over 2 million more require hospitalization as a result of proper pharmaceutical drug use.)

Most nutritional and herbal supplements on the market today also contain a single active ingredient. And while the risk of serious side effects, let alone death, caused by the use of nutritional and herbal supplements is extremely rare, the effectiveness of single ingredient supplements is often not as great as when the ingredients are obtained from food, along with their supporting co-factors.

For example, many people today are taking a vitamin B6 supplement to combat stress and/or to have more energy. While B6 can be beneficial for these purposes, it is more effective when obtained along with a full spectrum of B-complex vitamins, each of which works synergistically with the other members of the vitamin B family. Foods that are rich in B vitamins, such as beef, liver, eggs, nuts, and certain dark, leafy green vegetables, such as spinach, typically contain most or all of the B vitamins, along with various other B-supporting co-factors and other vitamins and minerals. Moreover, the B vitamins found in such foods are far more bio-available, meaning the body is better able to assimilate and make use of them than it is able to utilize synthetic B vitamin supplements.

This is but one example. The bottom line is that ongoing research in the fields of diet and nutrition continues to prove that Hippocrates was right: When it comes to our medicine, foods grown as nature intended really are our best choice.

Which brings me to coconuts. Few foods rank higher than coconut as a complete food source of essential vitamins (including B vitamins), minerals, proteins, carbohydrates, healthy fats, and fiber. This fact alone helps explain why coconuts have for centuries been a staple food in the tropical regions of the world in which coconuts are found.

Coconut water, the liquid found inside coconuts (which is not the same thing as commercial coconut water products, nor coconut milk, although the terms are often used interchangeably), is also rich in nutrients, including electrolytes. These elecrtolytes regulate the electric charge on your body's cells and the flow of water across their membranes, and also carry electrical impulses from the nerves that control your body's tissue function and movement. Electrolytes need to be replenished whenever we perspire heavily, making coconut water an ideal, refreshing drink following times of physical activity, especially in hot weather.

The rich nutritional profile of coconuts explains why coconut in all of its forms (meat, milk, water, oil, and flour) has in recent years caught the attention of researchers and physicians for its potential as a powerful health aid. I wrote this book to share their findings, so that you can discover for yourself the full array of health benefits coconuts can provide you. In the pages that follow, you will learn:

- The history of coconut use as a healing aid in the tropical regions of the world in which coconuts grow.

- The reasons why coconuts, as well as coconut water, milk, oil and flour, are so good for you.

- The healthy fats that coconuts contain and why they are so important to good health.

- How and why coconuts can protect your heart and improve blood pressure levels.

- The ways in which coconuts can aid healthy brain function and the promise it holds for helping to prevent, and even possibly reverse, dementia and Alzheimer's disease.

- How coconuts can boost your body's immune system and help fight infectious disease.

- Coconut's valuable benefits for healthy weight loss.

- Why adding coconuts and coconut oil to your diet can help banish fatigue and make a big, positive difference in your energy levels.

- How coconuts can help protect against diabetes.

- The uses coconuts and coconut oil have as a beauty aid and as an aid for healthy teeth and gums.

- Why coconut oil is one of the very best oils for your cooking and baking needs.

- Why coconut flour is valuable as an alternative to wheat flour now that so many people are suffering from gluten sensitivities.

And I'll also share with you what you need to know and look for when choosing and using coconut products, as well as the best sources for obtaining them.

So, if you are ready to discover the centuries-old healing secret of the tropics, keep reading.

1.

The Jewel of the Tropics

The Jewel of the Tropics

The Tree of Heaven

The Tree of Life

The Tree of Abundance

The King of Trees

The Tree of a Thousand Uses

What do all of the above names have in common? They are all traditional names for the coconut palm, and refer to the many benefits its fruit, the coconut, provides. So esteemed is the coconut palm in the countries in which it grows that, in India, the Sanskrit term for the coconut tree is *Kalpa Vriksha,* which means "the tree that gives all that is necessary for living." In Polynesia, it is said, "He who plants a coconut tree plants food and drink, vessels and clothing, a home for himself, and a heritage for his children."

During his travels through India, Sri Lanka, and southeast Asia, the thirteenth century explorer, Marco Polo, confirmed how valuable coconuts were in these regions. In a passage in *Travels,* the four book account of his

---

What Is a Coconut?

Technically speaking, the coconut palm is not actually a tree at all, since it is devoid of both bark and branches. It is actually a *monocotyledon,* or *monocot,* a species of flowering plants characterized by their seeds, which have only a single embryonic leaf, or *contyledon.* Contyledons are part of the embryos in seeds and are responsible for generating other parts of the plant. In addition to the coconut palm, other examples of moncotyledons include bamboo, sugar cane, and orchids.

famous journeys, he wrote "One of these nuts is a meal for man, both meat and drink." What he wrote, however, tells only part of the story about all of the benefits coconuts provide.

THE FRUIT WITH MANY USES

The scientific name for the coconut palm is *Cocos nucifera*. *Cocos* refers to its genus, while *nucifera* is a Latin term that means "nut-bearing." Though they may be considered nuts because of their name, botanically speaking, coconuts are actually a type of fruit known as a *drupe*, which translates to "stone fruit" and refers to any type of fleshy fruit with a hard covering that encloses a seed. Cherries, peaches, plums, and olives are also drupe fruits— the term *drupe* itself is derived from the word *drupa* (also *druppa*), which means "over-ripe olive."

Compared to other drupes, as well as fruits in general, coconuts are unrivaled when it comes to their versatility in terms of all of the benefits that they provide. In the West, this fact became known two centuries after Marco Polo wrote about coconuts, when his statement was echoed and elaborated upon by Antonio Pigafetta, a Venice nobleman who accompanied Fernando Magellan in the latter's expeditions to the East Indies.

In his journal, Pigafetta wrote:

> Coconuts are the fruit of the palm tree. And as we have bread and wine, oil and vinegar, so those people [the natives of the East Indies] get all these things from that tree. They get wine in the following manner. They bore a hole into the heart of the said palm at the top called palmito [stalk], from which distils a liquor which resembles white must [unfermented juice]. That liquor is sweet but somewhat tart, and [is collected] in [bamboo] canes as thick as the leg and thicker. They fasten the bamboo to the tree at evening for the morning, and in the morning for the evening.
>
> That palm bears a fruit, namely, the cocoanut, which is as large as the head or thereabouts. Its outside husk is green and thicker than two fingers. Certain filaments are found in that husk, whence is made cord for binding together their boats. Under that husk there is a hard shell, much thicker than the shell of the walnut, which they burn and make therefrom a powder that is useful to them. Under that shell there is a white marrowy substance one finger in thickness, which they eat fresh with meat and fish as we do bread; and it has a taste resembling the almond. It could be dried and made into bread. There is a clear, sweet water in the middle of that marrowy substance which is very refreshing. When that water stands for a while after having been collected, it congeals and becomes like an apple.

When the natives wish to make oil, they take that coconut, and allow the marrowy substance and the water to putrefy. Then they boil it and it becomes oil like butter. When they wish to make vinegar, they allow only the water to putrefy, and then place it in the sun, and a vinegar results like [that made from] white wine.

From the said fruit milk can also be made, as we proved by experience. For we scraped that marrow, then mixed it with its own water, and being passed through a cloth it became like goat's milk. This kind of palm tree is like the palm that bears dates, but not so knotty. And of these trees two will sustain a family of ten persons. But they do not draw the aforesaid wine always from one tree, but take it for a week from one, and so with the other, for otherwise the trees would dry up. And in this way they last one hundred years.

A HISTORY OF COCONUTS

The extensive history of coconuts rivals the versatility of its many uses. Because of its value both as a portable food and water source, the coconut played a central role in both the migration, colonization, and development of civilization in tropical regions of the Pacific and Indian Oceans.

The Traveling Fruit

Coconut palms grow on tropical islands all over the world, but the exact origin of the coconut is uncertain. It was long thought that coconuts first appeared in the islands located within the Indian and Pacific Oceans. Coconut fossil remnants dating back to the Eocence era, a period that began approximately 55 million years ago and ran for 18 million more years, have been found in both Australia and India. In recent years, some researchers have theorized that the fruit may have originally come from the Americas. For the most part, though, the Indo-Pacific origin remains the most likely.

Early forms of the coconut were well-suited for ocean dispersal, allowing the fruit to populate emerging islands of the coral atoll ecosystem. These coconuts did not look like the kind we are most familiar with today, however. In order to survive and spread across the sea, the original coconuts required a very thick husk to protect the seed they contained and had a slow germination time. They were also more angular and ridged in shape, with a pointed base that enabled them to take hold in the sand. It is speculated that these coconuts were able to be carried along the ocean currents for over a hundred days, across distances of as many as 3,000 miles, while still being able to germinate once they reached new land. For this reason, coconuts are sometimes referred to as a "dispersal fruit."

The Role of Coconuts in the Migration, Colonization, and Development of Civilization

Until humans intervened, coconuts were found only along the island coast, not inland. The primary carriers of coconuts to new lands were the Austronesian people, an ethnic population in parts of Asia, Oceania, and Africa. It is speculated that, beginning as early as 5,000 to 2,500 BCE, the Austronesians migrated and settled in lands that range from the Philippines to Malaysia to Polynesia. The origin of the Austronesians is uncertain; it was initially thought that they migrated from southeastern regions of modern-day China, but more recent evidence suggests that the spread of the Austronesian people may actually have begun from the regions of the Philippines and Taiwan. Whatever the case may be, it is known for certain that Austronesians had long been one of the world's most skilled seafaring peoples. The trade routes they traveled extend not only throughout lands in Pacific and Indian Oceans but also to parts of Africa and South America.

Interestingly, the genetic analysis of coconuts has, in part, confirmed the travel patterns of the Austronesians. Research has shown that there are two distinct genetic strains of domesticated coconuts: one that originated in the Indian Ocean, and another in the Pacific. But there is also evidence that both strains were mixed, with genetic material from each strain passing into the other. This mixed pattern coincides with the known trade routes of the Austronesians.

Many centuries after the Austronesians first began to migrate and trade across the lands of the Pacific and Indian Oceans, Spanish and Portuguese sailors traveling in those regions brought back coconuts to other lands, including parts of Mexico, the Caribbean, Arabia, and Turkey. In fact, it is thanks to these explorers that the name *coconut* exists today. It is derived from the Spanish and Portuguese term *coco*, which means "head" or "skull." The explorers used the term because of how the three characteristic indentations of coconuts resemble the features of a face. Prior to being called *coco*, the common term used for coconuts by Western explorers, including the famous British explorer Sir Francis Drake, was *nargils*. The term *coconut* itself did not come into common usage until the 1700s.

Coconuts are now grown in over ninety nations around the world, with over sixty tons, on average, harvested each year. More than 70 percent of the world's coconut supply comes from Indonesia, India, and the Philippines. Other lands in which coconuts are grown include Australia, Bermuda, parts of South America, Vietnam, Thailand, Saudi Arabia, and the United Arab Emirates. In addition to Hawaii, coconuts are also grown in parts of Florida.

Coconuts in Myth

The importance of coconuts to the peoples of the Pacific lands can be found in various creation myths from the region, which extend back through many centuries. One such myth comes from the Cook Islands, which are located in the South Pacific Ocean between French Polynesia and American Samoa. In the myth, the universe is said to be akin to a vast, hollow coconut shell. The outer surface of this shell is the upper world home of the mortals, while the shell's interior is the underworld. At the bottom of this shell there is said to be a thick stem that tapers off to a point. This stem represents the beginning of all things within creation and sustains the entire universe, in much the same way that the coconut palm and its fruit provide for most of the needs of the peoples of the region.

Similar creation myths can be found among the peoples of the Philippines. One myth holds that, at the beginning of creation, three gods ruled the universe: Bathala, the overseer of the earth; Ulilang Kaluluwa, the serpent snake who lived in the clouds; and Galang Kaluluwa, the winged god who traveled throughout the universe. According to the myth, the gods were initially unaware of each other. Bathala desired to create mortals on earth, but because the earth was barren, he was unable to do so. He was then visited by Ulilang Kaluluwa, who was angered to discover Bathala's existence. Wanting to be the sole ruler of the universe, he fought Bathala, but was killed by him after three days of battle, and Bathala buried his remains.

Sometime later, Galang Kaluluwa's travels brought him to earth where he, too, discovered Bathala. Rather than fighting each other, the gods became friends and remained so until Galang Kaluluwa's passing. Before it occurred, Galang Kaluluwa instructed Bathala to bury him beside the remains of Ulilang Kaluluwa, and Bathala did so.

From the grave of the two gods, a palm began to grow with a nut-shaped fruit. This was the coconut tree. Its appearance enabled Bathala to at last fulfill his dream of creating life on the earth, and so he created the first man and woman, along with all of the animals and vegetation. Using the trunk and leaves of the coconut palm, Bathala built a home for the man and woman, and to nourish them, he instructed them to drink the coconut water and eat its meat, and to use all of the palm to provide for their other needs. And so it was that life flourished across the earth.

These are but two examples of the creations myths in which the coconut plays a central role. Many others can also be found throughout the islands of the Pacific Ocean.

THE MULTIFACETED COCONUT

There are two distinct varieties of coconut: *niu kafa,* which is mostly used for producing fiber, rope, matting, and so forth, and *nui vai,* the domesticated form that is sold in grocery stores today. *Nui vai* coconuts are more suitable for eating, with a thinner husk and more meat and milk. They are more circular in form and are not as capable of remaining buoyant in the sea, as *niu kafa* coconuts are.

Coconuts have three distinct layers. The outermost layer is known as the *exocarp,* and is smooth, with a greenish color. The middle layer is known as the *mesocarp* and is composed of a fibrous husk that covers the hard, woody inner layer, or *endocarp.* Contained within the endocarp is the endosperm, which is part liquid—coconut water—and part solid—the white coconut flesh, or meat. The coconuts that you can buy in a store have both the exocarp and mesocarp layers removed, so what you are buying is the endocarp.

In addition to the benefits that coconuts provide as a food, milk, and oil, many other benefits can be supplied by coconuts and the palms on which they grow. What follows is an overview of some of these benefits.

Coconut Roots

Traditionally, coconut roots are used to make dyes. They can also be boiled to produce a natural remedy for various gastrointestinal problems, including dysentery and diarrhea. Small pieces of the root, when dried, can also be used to make toothbrushes.

Coconut Palm Trunks

If you travel through many of the regions in which the coconut palm grows, you will soon notice that many huts, houses, and other small buildings are constructed from the trunks of the palm. The trunks are ideal for these uses because of their strength and their resistance to salt from nearby seas. Many small bridges in these regions are also built from coconut palm trunks. The trunk has also traditionally been used to make canoes, as well as drums and various types of containers in many tropical regions. Timber supplied from the coconut palm is increasingly being used as a substitute for hardwoods derived from endangered trees.

Coconut Husks and Shells

The husks and shells of coconuts also have a number of important traditional uses. Due to their spherical shape, they are ready-made cups, bowls, and ladles. They can also be used to make buttons, a common feature of traditional Hawaiian shirts.

Coconuts Inspire New Research in the Design of Earthquake-Proof Buildings

In July 2016, the Society for Experimental Biology issued a press release stating that researchers at the Plant Biomechanics Group of the University of Freiburg, Germany are now studying coconuts for clues on how to best design buildings to resist damage caused by earthquakes. "Coconuts are renowned for their hard shells, which are vital to ensure their seeds successfully germinate. But the specialized structure of coconut walls could help to design buildings that can withstand earthquakes and other natural disasters," the release began.

The press release further noted that coconut palms can grow up to thirty meters in height (approximately ninety feet), and that when ripe coconuts fall from such a distance, their shells prevent them from splitting open when they hit the ground. It is because of their three-layered structure that coconuts are able to remain intact after impact and protect the seeds that they contain. According to the press release, the researchers are now working with civil engineers and material scientists to explore how this specialized coconut structure can be applied in architecture.

In order to survive the impacts of earthquakes and other natural disasters, buildings need to be able to effectively disperse energy, something coconuts are able to do extremely well. To determine how coconuts accomplish this, the researchers studied them using compression machines and an impact pendulum to analyze how coconuts react to impacts. They also employed microscopy and computer tomography to analyze the coconut shell's anatomy in order to "identify mechanically relevant structures for energy absorption." What the researchers discovered was that within the coconuts' inner layer, "the vessels that make up the vascular system have a distinct, ladder-like design, which is thought to help withstand bending forces. Each cell is surrounded by several lignified [woody] rings, joined together by parallel bridges."

Based on their findings, the researchers theorized that the distinct angle of the vascular bundles in the inner layer of coconuts could be modeled and applied to how textile fibers within functionally graded concrete are arranged, with the aim of better enabling crack deflection. As plant biomechanist Stefanie Schiemer explains, "this combination of lightweight structuring with high energy dissipation capacity is of increasing interest to protect buildings against earthquakes, rock fall, and other natural or human-made hazards."

In many tropical regions, the husks and shells are used as a fuel source and as a source of charcoal. The shell of the coconut is often used to manufacture activated charcoal, a highly effective agent for removing chemical impurities in manufacturing processes, such as metal finishing and electroplating, water purification, sewage treatment, and in the production of air filters in gas masks and respirators. Taken internally, the activated charcoal derived from coconut shells can also be used as an antidote for certain poisons and drug overdoses, as well as for relieving diarrhea, flatulence, and indigestion. It is likely this is the reason cups made from coconut shells have long been traditionally used to protect against poisoned drinks.

In tropical regions ranging from the Philippines to Jamaica, dried coconut husks and shells are used to brush and buff floors. In some cultures, the fresh, non-dried husk of brown coconuts can serve as a sponge. In Thailand, the husks are used to pot tree saplings. In regions where mosquitoes are common, such as southern India, coconut husks and shells are burned because the smoke they produce acts like a natural mosquito repellant.

In many regions of the world in which coconuts are grown—ranging from China, the Philippines, and Vietnam, to parts of Turkey and Saudia Arabia—the dried half shells of coconuts are used to make a variety of traditional musical instruments. In the West, coconut half shells are often banged together to produce sound effects such as the "clop clop" of a horse's hoof beats in radio and theatrical plays.

Coconut Fiber

The fiber from the husk of coconuts, which is called *coir*, has multiple uses. In many tropical regions, coir is used to make brushes, door mats, ropes, and sacks. In addition, it is used for caulking, including as a sealant for boats. Coir also makes a good fibrous stuffing in mattresses. In some cultures, coconut fiber is used to make compost for gardening purposes, particularly as an aid for growing orchids.

Coconut Oil

Coconut oil is produced by processing the *copra*, or dried meat of the coconut. In addition to its uses for cooking, coconut oil is a primary ingredient in many of the oil remedies used in Ayurveda, the traditional system of medicine from India. It can also be used to make soaps, hair conditioners and shampoos, skin moisturizers, toothpaste, and other cosmetic products (see Chapters 11 and 12).

Coconut Fronds

Coconut fronds, the ribbed coconut leaves of the coconut palm, are often used to make brooms and brushes. The green leaves are stripped away from the fronds' remaining veins, which are long, thin, and stiff, to produce the ends of brooms and brushes that are then attached to wooden handles.

Various parts of coconut fronds can also be used to make baskets, including water-tight baskets used to draw well water. Other uses for coconut fronds include making roofing thatch, mats, and cooking skewers. In countries such as Indonesia, Malaysia, and Singapore, small coconut fronds are often woven together to create a shell that is then filled with rice. The rice and the leaves are cooked together to make a traditional dumpling dish known as *ketupat.* And in India and other Asian countries, coconut fronds are used to make temporary shelters known as *pandals,* which are used for weddings and other ritual ceremonies in both Hindu and Buddhist traditions.

THE LONG HISTORY OF COCONUTS AS A HEALING AGENT

For thousands of years, the peoples of the Pacific and Indian Ocean lands have valued coconut as a useful folk medicine. Traditionally in these lands, coconut and its milk and oil have been used as a remedy for a wide range of health conditions, including bruising and minor burns, colds and flu, stomach upset and other gastrointestinal problems, and more.

The first extensive documentation of the various healing properties of coconuts can be found in the early writings of Ayurvedic medicine, or *Ayurveda.* Ayurveda, which means "life knowledge," is one of the world's oldest systems of medicine. Because of its broad scope, Ayurveda is often referred to as "the mother of all healing systems."

Ayurveda originated in ancient India and dates back at least 3,000 years. Two of its most ancient texts are the *Sushruta Samhita* and the *Charaka Samhita,* which are said to be written by the sage healers Sushruta and Charaka. respectively. Charaka is credited with the discovery that all substances, both organic and inorganic, as well as one's thoughts and actions, have definite potential or active attributes and can directly influence health and disease, making him one of the earliest proponents of what today is known as mind/body medicine.

Both the *Sushruta Samhita* and the *Charaka Samhita* discuss the value of coconut, including its oil, for healing. Among the many benefits attributed to coconut and its oil in the *Sushruta Samhita* are improved digestion; promotion of hair growth and improved quality and strength; nourishment of body tissues; healing of wounds; and natural coolant effects in and on the body. According to Sushruta, coconut and its oil can also be useful in the treatment of certain diseases, including malnutrition and emaciation, physical debility,

How Coconuts Helped Save the Life of a Future U.S. President

One of the most noteworthy uses of a coconut occurred during World War II. On August 1st, 1943, future U.S. President John F. Kennedy and his crew aboard PT-109 were shipwrecked near the Solomon Islands in the Pacific Ocean after colliding with a Japanese destroyer. Following the collision, Kennedy and his surviving crew members swam to safety to a tiny island known as Plum Pudding. Finding little to sustain them there, they swam to another island called Olasana. There, they foraged for food and drink, and were able to stay alive due to Kennedy's discovery of coconuts and fresh water.

Meanwhile, on the day of the collision, the explosion caused by the PT boat's impact with the destroyer was spotted by Sub-Lieutenant Arthur Reginald Evans from a watch post atop the island Kolombangara. Determining that the explosion was likely related to the now lost PT boat, on August 2nd, Evans dispatched two native islanders, Biuku Gasa and Eroni Kumana, to search for Kennedy and his crew. Eventually, the two natives discovered Kennedy and his men, but had trouble communicating with them due to a language barrier. In addition, their canoe was too small to safely transport Kennedy and all of his men.

The only solution was for Kennedy to write a message that the islanders could take back to the nearest Allied base. However, no one had paper or writing utensils. Gasa solved this problem by plucking a coconut from a nearby palm and instructing Kennedy to carve a message on the inside of its husk. Kennedy did so.

The message read, "Nauru Isl[and] commander / native knows posit[ion] / he can pilot / 11 alive need small boat / Kennedy." With the message in tow, Gasa and Kumana, at great risk to their own lives, rowed their canoe thirty-five miles to the Allied base at Rendova Island, from which was dispatched a rescue crew to bring Kennedy and his crew to safety.

Were it not for the presence of coconuts on the island of Olasana, John F. Kennedy's fate might have been very different. In gratitude for their heroic actions, Kennedy invited both Gasa and Kumana to attend his presidential inauguration. The coconut husk was eventually returned to him, and he kept it on his desk throughout his presidency. Today the husk can be found on display in the John F. Kennedy Library.

respiratory conditions, diabetes, and conditions of the bladder, kidney, and urinary tract.

As Ayurveda continued to develop, the healing properties of coconut milk and oil continued to be well-documented. In addition, coconut oil was found to be an essential ingredient for the preparation of other Ayurvedic remedies, both those taken internally and those applied externally. Such remedies were found to be useful for the treatment of dandruff, eczema and various other skin conditions, diseases related to the head and ears, rheumatism and other joint conditions, cramps, pain, and headache.

Many centuries before modern science confirmed that the fatty acid content of coconuts changes as they grow, Ayurvedic practitioners had already recognized the internal changes that occur as coconuts mature, and realized that these changes also result in different properties at different stages of coconuts' life cycle. For this reason, Ayurvedic texts divide coconuts into three distinct types: *baal*, or tender, young coconuts, *madhyam*, or half-mature (mid-stage) coconuts, and fully mature coconuts, known as *pakva*.

Baal coconuts are comprised of 90 to 95 percent water, or milk, which Ayurveda practitioners state is the most pure and most healing for purposes of cooling internal organs, healing the gastrointestinal tract, lubricating joints, and expelling toxins. *Madhyam*, or middle-stage coconuts have less water than *baal* coconuts, and its water is milkier. They are also characterized by their soft, pulpy meat, or flesh. The classical medical texts of Ayurveda state that when they are in their madhyam stage, coconuts are most nutritious. Modern research has confirmed this, finding that coconuts at this stage of their growth contain more carbohydrates, protein, vitamins—especially vitamins A, B, and C—and minerals, such as magnesium, phosphorus, and potassium, than during the younger and older stages of their growth.

Chakara wrote that both tender and mid-stage coconuts have *bringhan*, *snigdha*, *seetani*, *balyani*, and *madurani* properties, meaning that they increase the quantity and improve the quality of all seven *dhatus*, or tissues, in the body as identified by Ayurveda. (The seven *dhatus* are strikingly similar to the major body tissues identified by modern science. They are *rasa*, which corresponds to plasma, *rakta*, which corresponds to blood, *mamsa*, which corresponds to muscle tissue, *meda*, which corresponds to fat, *asthi*, which corresponds to bone, *majja*, which corresponds to bone marrow and nerves, and *shukra*, which corresponds to the body's reproductive fluids.)

Mature, or *pakva*, coconuts are not advised to be eaten by themselves, according to the tenets of Ayurveda, because of their firmer meat pulp and low water content. Instead, they should be combined with other ingredients, such as in chutneys (a dish prepared by grinding coconut meat and combining it with salt, chilies, and other spices), roasted chickpeas, or spices, such as cardamom, cinnamon, cloves, curcumin (turmeric), ginger, and mustard seeds.

Given how highly regarded the coconut is within the Ayurvedic system of healing, as well as how common it is in many regions of India, it is not surprising that coconut and its milk and oil are all staple ingredients in the cooking traditions of many parts of the Indian subcontinent. This is not only because of coconut's delicious taste, but also because of how coconuts are recognized by the people in the region to be one of the original health foods in the world.

CONCLUSION

In this chapter, you learned how truly beneficial coconuts and, indeed, all parts of the coconut palm, are to the peoples of the tropics. You learned of the important role coconuts played in sustaining the ocean travelers of centuries past, and also how they helped to open up trade between people of different lands and cultures. You also learned of the health benefits coconuts have for centuries provided for people throughout the lands of the Pacific and Indian Oceans. Finally, you discovered that people have recognized the health benefits of coconuts for thousands of years.

Now it's time to take a look at what modern science says about coconuts. Why exactly is this most versatile food so healthy for you? Chapter 2 will answer that question.

2.

Why Coconuts Are So Good for Your Health

As you learned in Chapter 1, coconuts are staple food items in the traditional diets of peoples throughout the lands of the Pacific and Indian Oceans. Coconuts are also one of the best food sources of many of the important nutrients that are essential for our health. In fact, the meat and the water of a medium-sized coconut supply the minimum daily requirements of nearly all of the protein, carbohydrates, healthy fats, and vitamins, minerals, and other nutrients needed for good health. This is perhaps one of the reasons why people in tropical regions have a low incidence of many of the chronic disease conditions that afflict us here in the West. Let's take a closer look.

THE NUTRITIONAL CONTENT OF COCONUTS

Coconuts are a primary food source and feature prominently as the main food dish in a number of tropic island cultures. It is not an exaggeration to say that the coconut may be a perfect food. Few foods, when eaten alone, are capable of sustaining human life as completely as coconuts can.

A medium-sized coconut supplies about 400 grams of coconut meat and, depending on whether it is tender or fully matured, between one to five ounces of coconut water. Combined, the meat and water of a coconut of this size contain less than 400 calories. Each serving of coconut meat provides a healthy supply of protein and amino acids, vitamins, minerals, dietary fiber, and healthy fats. All of these nutrients, with the exception of fiber, are also found in coconut oil, as well as in fresh coconut water.

What follows is an overview of the nutritional composition of coconuts.

AMINO ACIDS

Amino acids are the building blocks of your body's proteins. There are twenty different kinds in all, each with a different chemical structure that combine to determine a protein's unique function. Amino acids fall into one of three categories: *nonessential,* which are readily made by the body; *essential,* which must be obtained through the diet or, less ideally, as a supplement; and *conditional*, which are typically essential only in times of illness, injury, or stress. Coconuts are an excellent food source of many amino acids.

■ *Alanine*

Alanine is a nonessential amino acid, and plays a number of important roles in the body. Among its functions are helping to convert glucose into energy, aiding in the elimination of toxins from the liver, and protecting cells from becoming damaged during intense or prolonged aerobic activity.

■ *Arginine*

Arginine is a conditional amino acid used in the body to help maintain the health of the liver, boost the body's immune system, maintain blood sugar levels, and regulate hormones, including insulin, growth hormone, and the pituitary hormone vasopressin. Dietary supplementation is necessary during infancy, since the bodies of newborn babies are unable to produce their own supply of arginine. For these reasons coconut can be a healthy food for infants, as can coconut water.

Large concentrations of arginine are found in the skin. It plays a key role in the health of all the body's connective tissues, particularly the muscles, and helps maintain the health of joints. Research has also shown that arginine can improve circulation and aide in treating and protecting against various types of heart disease, including angina, coronary artery disease, and intermittent claudication. It also helps protect against both male and female impotence, as well as erectile dysfunction.

■ *Aspartic Acid*

Aspartic acid, or aspartate, helps to boost metabolism. It also plays an important role in the body's Krebs cycle, a process by which other amino acids and biochemicals are synthesized to create energy. Research has shown that aspartic acid increases both stamina and endurance levels in athletes. In addition, it helps transport minerals needed to form healthy RNA and DNA to the cells, as well as strengthening the immune system by increasing the production of immunoglobulins and antibodies.

Aspartic acid is sometimes used to treat fatigue and depression due to the vital role it plays in producing energy at the cellular level. It does this by transferring a substance called nicotinamide adenine dinucleotide (NADH) from the main body of the cell into its mitochondria, where it is used to generate adenosine triphosphate (ATP), the fuel that powers all cellular activity. It also aids mental and cognitive function by increasing concentrations of

NADH in the brain. There, NADH boosts the production of neurotransmitters and chemicals needed for normal mental functioning. Aspartic acid also helps eliminate excess toxins from the cells, especially ammonia, which is very damaging to the brain and nervous system, as well as the liver.

■ Cystine

Cystine is a nonessential amino acid. Because of its sulfur content, cystine aids in the formation and protection of healthy skin, hair, bones, and connective tissue. Cystine can also help boost the healing of burns and wounds and improve joint flexibility, including in cases of rheumatoid arthritis. It has also been shown to be effective for helping to break down and eliminate excess mucus in the lungs, and to protect against various types of respiratory conditions, including bronchitis and emphysema.

Cystine is needed by the body to produce *glutathione*, an antioxidant that protects against and helps repair free-radical damage. It works closely with glutathione to remove toxins from the liver and is often used in hospital emergency rooms to treat acetaminophen and other drug overdoses that are known to cause liver damage. It also protects the liver and brain against toxins absorbed from alcohol and cigarette use, and may help prevent hangovers.

■ Glutamic Acid

Glutamic acid, also called glutamate, is converted by the body into either glutamine or gamma-aminobutyric acid (GABA), two other amino acids that help transmit messages to the brain. Glutamate acts as a major excitatory neurotransmitter in both the brain and spinal cord. Excitatory neurotransmitters increase the firing of neurons in the central nervous system, causing an electrochemical impulse that nerve cells use to transmit signals. Research has shown that glutamic acid can help treat personality disorders, as well as childhood behavioral disorders. It can also be used to treat epilepsy, muscular dystrophy, ulcers, and hypoglycemic coma, a complication of insulin treatment for diabetes.

■ Glycine

Glycine plays many vital roles in keeping the body healthy. It is essential for maintaining healthy functioning of the central nervous and digestive systems and for the production of normal DNA and RNA strands—the genetic material needed for proper cellular formation and function. Glycine also helps to regulate blood sugar levels and is essential for proper functioning of the gastrointestinal tract, including digestion and the metabolizing of fats. In men, glycine can help maintain the health of the prostate gland and prevent and reduce symptoms of prostatic hyperplasia (BPH). It can also be useful for treating low energy and fatigue, such as hypoglycemia, anemia, and chronic fatigue syndrome (CFS).

High concentrations of glycine are found in the muscles, skin, and other connective tissues. It helps the body create and maintain healthy muscle tissue while preventing muscle breakdown. In addition, nearly one-third of collagen is composed of glycine. Collagen is essential for maintaining the firmness and flexibility of the skin and connective tissue. The body uses glycine to repair damaged tissues, heal wounds, and to protect against ultraviolet (UV) rays from sunlight, oxidation, and free radical damage.

Research has shown that glycine can help inhibit the neurotransmitters in the brain that can trigger seizures, hyperactivity, and manic (bipolar) depression. Additional research indicates that it may be beneficial for managing the symptoms of schizophrenia. It can also protect against memory loss, particularly memory loss caused by lack of sleep, jet lag, and overwork.

■ Histadine

Histadine is needed to produce and maintain healthy tissues throughout the body, especially myelin sheaths. These sheaths coat nerve cells and without them the transmission of messages from the brain to other parts of the body could not occur. Researchers have found that histidine acts as a detoxifying agent in the body, and can protect against damage caused by radiation. It also aids in the elimination of heavy metals in the body, and is crucial for the production of both red and white blood cells, thereby aiding immune function.

■ Isoleucine

Isoleucine's primary function in the body is to boost energy, increase endurance, and aid in the recovery from strenuous physical activity. It is involved in the production of healthy clotting injury sites in the body, and also plays a vital role in the healing and repair of muscle tissue. Isoleucine keeps energy levels stable by helping to maintain blood sugar levels. Because of its ability to regulate blood sugar, it helps protect against symptoms associated with low blood sugar (hypoglycemia), including "brain fog" and confusion, depression, dizziness, fatigue, headaches, and irritability.

Isoleucine also acts as one of three branched-chain amino acids (BCAAs). The two other BCAAs are leucine and valine. Together, BCAAs help promote muscle health and repair and supply energy to muscle tissue.

■ Leucine

Leucine is the most effective BCAA for preventing muscle loss, and also highly effective for improving the healing of bones, skin, and muscle tissue caused by injury. Leucine also helps to regulate blood sugar and, like isoleucine, protects against symptoms associated with low blood sugar. It is also used by the body to increase the production of growth hormone, and helps to burn visceral fat, or fat located in the deepest layers of the body that is most resistant to both dieting and exercise.

■ *Lysine*

Lysine is an essential amino acid best known for its ability to enhance the body's immune system and to help produce antibodies that protect against infection, especially from viruses. Lysine is particularly useful for protecting against herpes viruses, as well as cold sores and shingles. In addition, it is required for proper hormone production and bone growth and overall bone health in both children and adults. It also plays a role in the production of collagen and muscle tissue.

■ *Methionine*

Methionine is another essential amino acid that plays an important role in helping the body, especially the liver, process and eliminate fat. Like cystine, methionine also contains sulfur, which the body needs to produce glutathione, a powerful antioxidant, as well as the amino acids cysteine and taurine, both of which aid in the elimination of toxins, protect the cardiovascular system, and help to build healthy tissues. Methionine is essential for healthy skin, nails, and connective tissue due to the role it plays in the body's production of collagen.

■ *Phenylalanine*

Phenylalanine, another essential amino acid, plays a crucial role in helping to maintain normal functioning of the brain and central nervous system (CNS). Its effectiveness in this regard has to do with its ability to cross the blood-brain barrier, something that few nutrients are capable of doing. The blood-brain barrier is designed to protect the brain from toxins, bacteria, viruses, and other harmful microorganisms. Because of phenylalanine's ability to penetrate this barrier, it is able to directly and positively affect brain function. As a result, it has been found to be helpful for preventing and relieving conditions associated with impaired functioning of both the brain and CNS. Phenylalanine is also required by the body to produce the neurotransmitters epinephrine, dopamine, and norepinephrine, each of which plays an important role that affects how we perceive and interact with our external environment.

Research has shown that phenylalanine helps to improve mood, enhance memory and other cognitive functions, and reduce food cravings. It has also been shown to boost melatonin production, which is essential for healthy sleep. Additional research has found that phenylalanine can help ease symptoms of arthritis, anxiety and depression, and menstrual cramps, as well as helping to reverse obesity because of its ability to regulate appetite.

■ *Proline*

Proline plays an important role in the production of both cartilage and collagen. It helps muscles and joints maintain their flexibility, contributes to healthy skin tone, and protects against wrinkling. Proline is also used by the body to create healthy cells from proteins. It is crucial for the growth and maintenance of healthy skin and connective tissues, and also helps to repair these tissues when they become damaged by injuries. Research shows that proline helps improve recovery from exercise, prevents loss of muscle mass, and boosts endurance during times of strenuous activity. It has also been shown to benefit people suffering from osteoarthritis, chronic back pain, and muscle strain.

■ *Serine*

Serine plays a major role in the maintenance of both overall physical and mental health. It helps the body produce the phospholipids that in turn are needed to create every type of cell in the human body. Serine also aids in the functioning of RNA and DNA, and the metabolism of fat and fatty acids. In addition, serine is necessary for proper functioning of the brain and CNS. Both brain proteins and the myelin sheath that covers and protect nerves contain serine. Without enough serine, the myelin sheath can begin to fray, leading to impaired signaling between the brain and the nerves.

Serine helps produce antibodies and immunoglobulin, making it necessary for optimal immune function. It enhances the absorption of creatine, as well, thereby improving the body's ability to build and maintain muscle. It is also required in order for the body to produce tryptophan. Because of its role in tryptophan production, serine can help relieve symptoms of anxiety, depression, and insomnia. Research has also found that low levels of serine can be one of the factors that cause both chronic fatigue syndrome and fibromyalgia.

■ *Threonine*

Threonine, another essential amino acid, performs a number of vital functions in the body. By helping to maintain the proper balance of protein, it helps ensure normal growth of muscles and tissues. It also also helps both muscles and connective tissues remain strong and elastic, especially in the heart, where high concentrations of threonine are found. Threonine works with aspartic acid and methionine to maintain the liver's ability to metabolize fats and fatty acids. Lack of threonine makes it possible for fats to build up in the liver, causing fatty liver disease, and even liver failure.

Threonine also helps maintain the health and functioning of the central nervous system, where it is also found in high concentrations. It also helps increase the supply of glycine in the CNS, and, because it does so, research indicates threonine can be helpful for preventing and treating multiple sclerosis (MS) and other conditions that affect nerve and muscle function. It also plays a role in maintaining healthy immune function by aiding the body's production of antibodies.

■ *Tryptophan*

Tryptophan is best known for its ability to produce the hormone serotonin. Healthy serotonin levels enhance well-being, while lack of serotonin has been linked to anxiety, depression, irritability, mood swings, and other unhealthy emotions. Tryptophan also helps maintain proper signaling between nerve cells, and to produce various proteins, as well as vitamin B3 (niacin) and the hormone melatonin, which is essential for healthy sleep.

Research indicates that adequate tryptophan levels in the body can help prevent and alleviate a number of health conditions, ranging from bruxism (grinding of teeth) and facial pain, to attention deficit and attention deficit hyperactivity disorders (ADHD), anxiety, depression, and insomnia and other sleep disorders. Because of its calming effect, tryptophan can also be helpful as an aid to quitting smoking.

■ *Tyrosine*

Tyrosine is the final amino acid found in coconut. Tyrosine produces vital brain chemicals that control appetite and the body's responses to stress and pain. It also helps to regulate mood and maintain the overall functioning of the nervous system.

Tyrosine is necessary for the proper functioning of the adrenal, pituitary, and thyroid glands, and for maintaining healthy metabolism. Lack of tyrosine can cause metabolism to become sluggish, and also contribute to chronic fatigue, hypothyroidism, low blood pressure, and low libido. In addition, tyrosine is used by the body in combination with phenylalanine to produce the neurotransmitters dopamine, epinephrine, and norepinephrine, which impact how we perceive and interact with our external environment. Without enough tyrosine, the body cannot produce its own supply of phenylalanine. Conversely, without enough phenylalanine, the body cannot produce its own supply of tyrosine. Coconut supplies the body with both of them.

VITAMINS

Coconuts also supply a number of important vitamins.

■ *Vitamin B1*

Vitamin B1, or thiamine, is a crucial nutrient needed to maintain the proper functioning of both the brain and nervous system. Like all other B vitamins, it is water-soluble, meaning that it must be replenished daily from vitamin B-rich foods or nutritional supplementation. B vitamins are eliminated from the body through urination and sweating, and their supply in the body can also be diminished in response to stress.

Thiamine is necessary in order for foods, especially carbohydrates, to be converted into energy once they are consumed. This energy conversion occurs in part because of how the body uses B1 to produce a substance called thiamin pyrophosphate (TPP). Without TPP, the body cannot convert food into energy. In addition, thiamine helps to protect the muscles of the heart and keep them healthy and helps to regulate heart beat.

■ *Vitamin B2*

Vitamin B2, or riboflavin, plays a variety of important roles in the body. It regulates red blood cell growth and boosts immune function by protecting the body from free-radical damage. B2 is also responsible for maintaining the health of hair, nails, and skin, as well as healthy vision. In addition, riboflavin helps to improve memory and supports healthy brain function.

Like B1, B2 is also necessary for the conversion of food into energy. It does this by producing two enzymes, known, respectively, as flavin mononucleotide and flavin adenine dinucleotide. Both are necessary to convert proteins, carbohydrates, and fats into energy. B2 is also needed in order for other B vitamins, especially vitamins B3 and B6, to properly perform their functions.

■ *Vitamin B3*

Vitamin B3, or niacin, works in conjunction with other B vitamins to produce and release energy in the cells, and to maintain proper functioning of the nervous system. Niacin is also responsible for proper circulation in the body, as well as for regulating blood sugar levels and the production of hormones. Research has also shown that niacin is helpful for preventing and treating a wide range of health conditions, including canker sores, circulatory problems, depression, digestive problems, fatigue, inflammation, insomnia, low blood sugar, muscle cramps, PMS, and tinnitus. It also helps to maintain healthy skin.

One of B3's most important functions is its ability to maintain healthy levels of both HDL and LDL cholesterol. This fact was proven by research conducted in the 1950s by Dr. Abram Hoffer and two-time Nobel Laureate Linus Pauling, who found that supplementation of vitamin B3 boosted levels of HDL ("good") cholesterol while simultaneously lowering levels of LDL ("bad") cholesterol. Unlike cholesterol drugs, especially statin drugs, B3 provides these important health benefits without causing any side effects.

■ Vitamin B5

Vitamin B5, or pantothenic acid, is one of the most useful vitamins for preventing and combating stress, as well as anxiety and depression. It is also needed to produce hormones, antibodies in the immune system, and healthy red blood cells. Like other B vitamins, it also aids the body in converting foods, especially carbohydrates and fats, into energy.

B5 is used by the body to produce coenzyme A, a substance that helps the body's detoxification processes and aids in the elimination of residues from drugs, as well as herbicides, insecticides, and other environmental toxins. B5 has also been shown to help boost energy and stamina because of how it supports the body's adrenal glands.

B5 helps support healthy skin and is useful for healing cuts and mild burns. In fact, a type of pantothenic acid known as *panthoderm* is commonly found in many commercial skin creams and lotions, which helps to explain why coconuts and coconut oils are also excellent for maintaining a healthy complexion (see Chapter 10).

■ Vitamin B6

Vitamin B6, or pyridoxine, has many uses in the body, including helping to convert foods into energy, boosting immune function, and maintaining the health of the nervous system. Pyridoxine also helps prevent the formation of unhealthy blood clots that can trigger both heart attack and stroke. It helps maintain healthy blood circulation and helps regulate hormone production. Pyridoxine can also help prevent and reverse varicose veins, and help minimize symptoms of carpal tunnel syndrome, diabetes, and PMS.

B6 is also an essential nutrient for protecting against heart disease due to its ability, in combination with vitamins B9 (folic acid) and B12, to break down and prevent the formation of homocysteine. Elevated homocysteine levels are a major risk factor for atherosclerosis (hardening of the arteries), heart disease, and stroke because it attracts cholesterol and causes it to be deposited within the arteries and muscles of the heart.

■ *Vitamin B9*

Vitamin B9, or folic acid, also plays a crucial role for energy production, and is necessary for the overall health of all of the body's cells. It also plays a vital role in the body's growth processes, beginning with the development of the fetus, making it an essential vitamin for women during pregnancy and breastfeeding. In addition, folic acid helps to boost immune function, regulates the production of both red and white blood cells, and is involved in the production of both DNA and RNA. It also helps maintain the health of the gastrointestinal tract, as well as the skin, the cells that line the small intestine, and red and white blood cells. Folic acid helps to form the DNA and RNA in our genes, which are needed to regulate cell formation.

■ *Vitamin C*

Vitamin C is one of the most versatile and important nutrients that the body needs. It is a powerful antioxidant essential for maintaining healthy tissues, repairing damaged tissues, protecting against cancer, and boosting overall immune function. It also plays a vital role in protecting the heart and overall cardiovascular system, maintaining optimal levels of collagen in the skin, and ensuring the health of bones, gums, and teeth.

Vitamin C also acts as a potent anti-inflammatory agent, thereby protecting and helping to reverse a wide range of health conditions, including arthritis, respiratory conditions, diabetes, fibromyalgia, joint pain, and sprains. In addition, research shows that vitamin C helps maintain the health of the eyes, and can help prevent cataracts, eyestrain, glaucoma, and other vision problems. It has also been shown to be helpful for preventing and relieving constipation, hangover, infertility, rashes, shingles, skin wrinkling, and sunburn. Because of its strong anti-bacterial and anti-viral properties, vitamin C is also an important nutrient for preventing and combating a wide range of infectious diseases, ranging from colds and flu to gastrointestinal infections, yeast infections, and urinary tract infections.

Vitamin C is water-soluble and cannot be produced by the body, so it must be replenished on a daily basis through the diet or, if necessary, as a nutritional supplement.

■ *Vitamin E*

Vitamin E is another important antioxidant that neutralizes free-radical damage. Vitamin E plays a crucial role in protecting the immune system, primarily because of its ability to increase levels of the interferon and interleukin, two biochemicals that are required by the immune system to prevent and fight off infections. Research has shown that adequate vitamin E levels in the body can help protect against a variety of other conditions as well, including certain types of cancer, respiratory conditions, various eye problems, including macular degeneration and vision issues related to diabetes, prostate enlargement, osteoarthritis, and sunburn. It has also shown promise for preventing Alzheimer's disease and dementia.

▇ *Vitamin K*

Vitamin K also plays a variety of important roles in the body. One of the most vital is its ability to produce various blood-clotting factors in the body that are necessary to prevent unchecked bleeding or hemorrhaging. Vitamin K is also necessary to maintain the health of the capillaries and helps to protect against and heal bruises and nosebleeds.

In addition, vitamin K helps to keep bones strong and healthy by enhancing their ability to absorb and store calcium. Studies have shown that lack of vitamin K can increase the risk of bone diseases such as osteoporosis, while also reducing the risks of bone and hip fractures. In part, this is due to how it prevents vitamin D from causing excess calcium to be displaced into the arteries and kidneys, thus reducing the risk of atherosclerosis, kidney stones, and other types of kidney disease associated with excess calcium buildup. Recently, researchers have also begun to study vitamin K's potential for reducing the risk of cancerous tumors.

MINERALS

Now that you know what vitamins coconuts contain, let's turn our attention to their mineral content.

Minerals are one of the most vital, yet overlooked class of nutrients. They play many essential roles in your body, and work in combination with vitamins, hormones, enzymes, and various other nutrient cofactors, to regulate thousands of biological functions. However, unlike various vitamins and other nutrients, your body cannot produce minerals on its own because they are inorganic nutrients. Therefore, it is crucial that you obtain an optimal supply of essential minerals each and every day. Eating coconuts, drinking fresh coconut milk and water, and using coconut oil are ways that you can do so.

Minerals and vitamins work synergistically, meaning that both classes of nutrients must be present in the body before either can perform their many functions. It is accurate to say that minerals act as catalysts for vitamins, and vice versa. Minerals and vitamins are also necessary in combination for the body to be able to produce various enzymes that are also essential for optimal health.

Most people today are deficient in at least some of the minerals that are essential for good health. This has been the case for decades here in the United States, in large part due to the mineral deficiencies in the soil in which food crops are raised. Such deficiencies have been caused by commercial farming methods which, unlike traditional farming practices, do not rotate crop production on an annual basis, and engage in the heavy use of pesticides, herbicides, and other substances that further deplete the mineral content in soil. Without an adequate supply of minerals, crops suffer from deficiencies in vitamins, minerals, and other nutrients. Lack of minerals in our food supply is one of the primary causes of our nation's still-expanding healthcare crisis. As Linus Pauling once said, "Lack of minerals is the cause of all disease."

The minerals found in coconut are as follows.

■ Calcium

Calcium is best known for its importance for building and maintaining strong bones, teeth, and connective tissue, but it plays other important roles in the body, as well. Among them are aiding digestion by producing enzymes involved in the digestive process, assisting in healthy blood clotting, and regulating the nerve impulses that signal muscles, including muscles of the heart, to contract. Research indicates that calcium can also help prevent high blood pressure and may reduce the risk of developing colon cancer. Although calcium supplements are a popular way for people to ensure they meet their bodies' calcium needs, a growing body of evidence is showing that the best way to obtain calcium is through food.

■ Copper

Copper also plays a variety of roles in the body, including helping to regulate and protect the cardiovascular and nervous systems. Copper is useful for maintaining bone health in the overall skeletal system, and helps protect against rheumatoid arthritis, osteoporosis. and joint pain. In addition, it is used in the body to produce phospholipids, the substances that are a component of all cell membranes, and which form the myelin sheaths that cover and protect nerves. Copper is also necessary to protect against atherosclerosis and to prevent arteries from rupturing. It can help protect against aneurysms and heart arrythmias, as well, and is also necessary for keeping blood properly oxygenated and for regulating blood pressure levels.

The body also uses copper to produce superoxide dismutase (SOD). Found in all living cells, SOD acts as a powerful antioxidant that protects cells, tissues, and organs from free radical damage. Copper also plays a role in maintaining the health of skin and hair, and is also used by the body to create melanin, the pigment that gives skin, hair, and eyes their color.

Iron

Iron is required for the production of hemoglobin in red blood cells, and works synergistically with copper in this process. Hemoglobin transports oxygen throughout the body, and gives red blood cells their color. Copper assists in the process by properly storing and releasing the body's iron stores when hemoglobin is produced. Iron deficiencies can lead to anemia, a condition characterized by fatigue, shortness of breath, and pale skin caused by a lack of oxygen. Iron also helps supply muscles with oxygen so that they can contract and function properly.

Magnesium

Magnesium is quite possibly the most important mineral required for optimal health. Primarily acting within the cells, magnesium is responsible for the proper functioning of approximately 80 percent of the body's metabolic processes. It does this by activating more than a thousand metabolic pathways in the body, including those responsible for protein, carbohydrate, and fat metabolism. Magnesium also plays a vital role in energy metabolism because it is essential for the production and functioning of adenosine triphosphate (ATP), the cells' main source of energy generation. Magnesium is also the essential nutrient for muscles, playing a vital role in their proper functioning and, most importantly, their relaxation. Without magnesium your muscles literally could not operate the way nature intended.

One of magnesium's most important functions is supporting the heart and overall cardiovascular system. Magnesium is also absolutely vital for proper heart function, and plays a crucial role in protecting against heart disease, including heart attacks, stroke and hypertension (high blood pressure). Research shows that magnesium acts as a natural calcium channel blocker, but without any of the health risks posed by calcium channel blocker drugs, and also helps to prevent the formation of dangerous blood clots. And its role in ATP production is also essential for protecting the heart, since heart muscle cells contain very high concentrations of mitochondria that depend on ATP to do their job. In addition, magnesium helps dilate blood vessels, making it easier for the heart to pump blood and more effectively transmit nutrients and oxygen to the body's cells, tissues, and organs.

Among its many other functions, magnesium enhances immune function and helps protect against infection, copies and repairs DNA, and aids in proper cell division, cell maintenance, and cell repair. It also acts as a "gatekeeper" for the cells by modulating the electrical potential across cell membranes. This, in turn, enables nutrients to enter into cells and cellular waste products to be excreted. One of the primary ways in which magnesium helps to accomplish this task is by regulating the cells' sodium/potassium pump, an active transport system that is responsible for ensuring that cells contain relatively high concentrations of potassium ions but low concentrations of sodium ions. When this ratio of high potassium to low sodium ions within the cells and high sodium to low potassium ions outside the cells is disturbed, the stage is set for disease to occur at the cellular level of the body.

Magnesium also protects against the accumulation of environmental toxins in the cells and tissues, and helps the body produce glutathione, a powerful antioxidant that protects against free radical damage and toxicity. It helps to activate and regulate hormones, as well, including helping to maintain proper functioning of the thyroid gland and other endocrine organs. It also regulates nerve function, and, along with calcium, is essential for healthy bones and teeth. And it prevents unhealthy calcium buildup (calcification) in the arteries and inside the kidneys, as well as regulating blood sugar levels.

■ Manganese

Manganese acts as an antioxidant, helping to prevent free radical damage. It also plays a role in maintaining healthy digestion, and helps the body convert fats and protein into energy. In addition, manganese helps bones grow and stay healthy and is useful for preventing and relieving osteoporosis. Among its other functions are helping to prevent and reduce fatigue levels, helping to regulate blood sugar levels, helping to improve thyroid function, and improving the functioning of the immune, nervous, and reproductive systems. It also plays a role in normal blood clotting, and it is needed for the body's production of cartilage and fluids in the joints that keep them lubricated. Manganese also helps the body absorb vitamin B1 and vitamin E, and works with all B vitamins to help prevent and relieve anxiety, depression, and other nervous disorders.

■ Phosphorus

Phosphorus is found in every cell of the body, but it is most abundant in bones and teeth, where it plays an essential role in their proper formation.

It also helps the body metabolize carbohydrates and fats, and is involved in the growth, maintenance, and repair of cells and tissues. Like magnesium, phosphorus also helps the body produce ATP, and, like manganese, it works synergistically with all B vitamins. It also helps maintain healthy heartbeat, kidney function, muscle contractions, and proper nerve signaling.

▓ *Potassium*

Potassium acts as an electrolyte, meaning that it helps electricity flow through your body. Most potassium in your body is found inside of your cells, but it moves outside of cell walls if necessary, in order to keep fluid steady in and around cells. This process, known as cellular membrane potential, is heavily regulated by your body in order to properly govern and sustain healthy electrical flow for the rhythm of your heartbeat. In addition, potassium is required for healthy nerve and muscle function and for maintaining proper blood pressure and blood sugar levels.

Lack of potassium in the body can result in a number of health problems, including a condition known as *hypokalemia*, which is caused when potassium is rapidly depleted from the body faster than it can be replenished, such as what happens with prolonged vomiting, diarrhea, and the overuse of diuretics. Symptoms of potassium deficiency include fatigue, muscle cramps and fatigue, bloating, constipation, abdominal pain, acne, depression, edema, nervousness, insatiable thirst, high cholesterol, insomnia, nausea, problems breathing, and sodium (salt) retention.

▓ *Selenium*

Selenium is an essential trace mineral that works well with vitamin E. Together, these two nutrients enhance each other's beneficial effects in the body, especially with regard to protecting against free radical damage. On its own, selenium is also used by the body to produce glutathione, as well as antioxidant enzymes known as *selenoproteins.* As a result, selenium has been shown by research to help reduce the risk of both cancer and heart disease, as well as arthritis. Additionally, selenium helps to boost immune function and, in men, can increase fertility.

▓ *Sodium*

Sodium (salt) has been demonized in recent decades as something that should be avoided. In truth, however, sodium is another important electrolyte. It is vital for the health of the body's extracellular fluid, and is an essential part of the cells' sodium/potassium pump. Sodium also plays an essential role in various enzyme functions in the body and is required for regulating the body's other fluids. It supports healthy muscle contraction, as well as helping to maintain the cardiovascular and nervous systems. Without sodium, your body would not be able to properly generate and transmit electrical impulses. Sodium also supports the health of the adrenal glands, and aids in glucose absorption.

Your body's sodium stores can become depleted when you sweat profusely or stay out in the sun too long in hot weather. Signs of sodium deficiency include confusion, diarrhea, dizziness, fatigue, headache, low blood pressure, muscle pain, and weakness.

■ Zinc

Zinc is another important mineral with many important functions in the body. Not only does zinc act as a potent antioxidant, it is also crucial for the health of the thymus gland and for the health of the immune system, especially with regard to the production of T-cells. Zinc also enhances digestion and helps maintain the health of the reproductive system, especially in men, due to its ability to boost the production of growth hormones and testosterone.

Research has shown that zinc can be effective for preventing and relieving a variety of health conditions, including acne, arthritis, colds and flu, canker sores, fibromyalgia, hemorrhoids, lupus, and macular degeneration. Zinc is needed for healthy bones, hair, skin, and nails, and can be an effective treatment for various skin conditions, such as eczema, rosacea, and psoriasis. It also helps maintain the health of the eyes (especially the retina) and ears, and can help prevent tinnitus.

FIBER

Carbohydrates are also a component of coconuts. Very little of their carbohydrate content is digestible however, making coconuts an ideal food for people who follow a low-carbohydrate diet. Most of the carbohydrates in coconuts (over 70 percent) are non-digestible. Non-digestible carbohydrates are better known as dietary fiber.

The standard American diet is very deficient in dietary fiber; studies reveal that it supplies no more than a third of the fiber necessary for optimal health, and in many cases, even less than that amount. Yet research clearly documents that a high-fiber diet is vital to good health. Studies of the dietary habits of people all around the world have shown that cultures that follow a high fiber diet typically have a much lower incidence of degenerative diseases. This is not surprising, given that research has also demonstrated that high dietary fiber intake can significantly reduce the risk of many serious health conditions, including heart disease, high blood pressure, certain types of cancer (especially colon and rectal cancer), type 2 diabetes, and gallbladder disease. High fiber diets also help prevent constipation, as well as hemorrhoids. Fiber-rich foods also support healthy gastrointestinal function and reduce the risk of a number of GI diseases, including colitis, diverticulitis, and irritable bowel syndrome (IBS). High fiber diets can also help aid people who are overweight or obese because of fiber's ability to satisfy hunger cravings.

Coconut meat is one of the world's richest sources of dietary fiber. A typical serving of coconut meat—one cup, or approximately eighty grams—on average provides twelve grams of fiber. This goes a long way toward meeting your daily fiber requirements, which is ideally thirty-five grams per day. Additionally, the dietary fiber in coconut meat has no calories, since fiber, by its very nature, is not absorbed by the body. Instead, it is used by the body to improve the removal of waste matter in the GI tract. It also absorbs and binds with toxins in the body, aiding in their elimination as well. For all of these reasons, adding coconut meat to your diet is an ideal way to not only help meet your daily dietary fiber requirements, but it is also one more way that coconuts can boost your overall health. Best of all, unlike various other fiber-rich foods, and certainly fiber supplements, coconut has the added benefit of being delicious.

FATS

The primary component in coconuts is fat, especially saturated fat, which makes up nearly 30 percent of coconuts' overall nutritional content. Coconuts also contain minute amounts of both monounsaturated and polyunsaturated fats.

Given coconuts' high saturated fat content, you may be asking yourself how coconuts can be regarded as a healthy food choice. Aren't saturated fats bad for our health?

For decades that has been the commonly accepted belief, including by most doctors and the medical establishment. The fact of the matter, however, is that belief is erroneous. What researchers now know is that saturated fats, especially the types of saturated fats coconuts contain, are actually very healthy for you, and a lack of such fats in your diet can result in serious unhealthy consequences.

Fully understanding the facts about fats, both good and bad, requires a full discussion that separates the myths about fats from the truth. You can find that discussion in the next chapter. For now, let me simply stress that the specific type of saturated fats that coconuts contain are one of the primary reasons why coconuts are indeed so healthy for you.

CONCLUSION

In this chapter, you learned about all of the important nutrients coconuts provide. Few foods contain such an abundance of nutrients, which is why coconuts are rightly regarded as one of the healthiest food choices you can make. In Chapter 3, you will learn even more reasons why coconuts are so good for your health, all of which have to do with their fat content. The information you will discover there may surprise you, so read on.

3.

Healthy Saturated Fats

As you learned in Chapter 2, fat, specifically saturated fat, and coconut oil are the two largest nutritional components of coconuts. To a lesser extent, saturated fats are also found in coconut milk and water. So how, you might ask, can coconuts and their oil, milk, and water possibly be good for your health? Aren't fats, especially saturated fats, unhealthy? No, they are not.

In fact, the type of saturated fats found in coconuts are very good for your health. As I mentioned in Chapter 2, researchers now know that saturated fats are indeed an important dietary contributor to good health. This chapter explains why this is so, and also explores how and why saturated fats have for so long been demonized as something to be avoided.

TYPES OF FATS

The three main classifications of dietary fats are saturated fats, unsaturated fats, and trans fats.

Saturated fats are also sometimes referred to as solid fats due to the fact that they remain solid at room temperature. They are primarily found in animal food products, especially meats, butter, cheese, milk, and other dairy products, but they are also derived from tropical plants, such as coconuts, palm fruits, and cocoa beans.

There are two types of unsaturated fats: monosaturated and polysaturated. These kinds of fats are liquid at room temperature. Monounsaturated fats are primarily found in nuts, seeds, and certain legumes, such as peanuts, as well as avocados and olives. Polyunsaturated fats, or PUFAs, are mainly found in vegetable oils, such as canola, corn, flaxseed, sesame, safflower, soybean, and sunflower oils, as well as in seafood.

Polyunsaturated fats are further divided into two separate classes of fatty acids: omega-3 fatty acids, which are found mainly in seafood and flaxseeds, and omega-6 fatty acids, which are primarily found in most other vegetable oils. A third form of omega fatty acid, known as omega-9, is primarily found in canola oil.

Trans fats, also called partially hydrogenated fats, are fats that are not found in nature. Instead, they are created through the process of *hydrogenation*, which involves combining hydrogen with fat compounds. The hydrogenation process makes trans fats harder and more solid at room temperature than saturated fats, and also extends their shelf life compared to other fats. However, trans fats are known to be unhealthy and should be entirely avoided. Although trans fats are increasingly being removed from commercial food products, they can still be found in many processed foods, snack foods such as chips and crackers, store-bought cookies, margarine, and commercial salad dressings.

A Question of Atoms

The difference between what makes a fat saturated rather than unsaturated all comes down to atoms. Specifically, carbon and hydrogen atoms. All types of fats or, more accurately, the fatty acids that make up fats, are composed of chains of carbon atoms. Each of these carbon atoms can hold, or have attached to it, up to two hydrogen atoms. Fatty acids in which two hydrogen atoms are attached to each carbon atom make up saturated fats. Saturated, in this context, means that each carbon atom has reached the limit of hydrogen atoms it can hold. In other words, it is *saturated* with hydrogen atoms.

Unsaturated fats contain carbon atoms chains that are missing one or more hydrogen atoms. Monounsaturated fats lack only pair of hydrogen atoms, while polyunsaturated fats lack more than two. The more hydrogen atoms missing from its carbon chain, the more polyunsaturated the fatty acid is said to be. When hydrogen atoms are missing from the carbon atoms in fatty acids, the carbon atoms form a double bond with each other. Monounsaturated fats have a single double bond, while polyunsaturated fats have more than one double bond. These double bonds can be considered "weak links" in the fatty acids' carbon chains.

Interestingly, the only oils that can be used to manufacture trans, or partially hydrogenated, fats are unsaturated fats. The reason for this is because saturated fats do not contain double bonds. Only fats with double bonds can be artificially reconfigured, which is precisely what happens to unsaturated fats during the manufacturing process that creates trans fats.

THE CHOLESTEROL MYTH

Until recently, unsaturated fats were touted as the healthiest type of dietary fat over saturated fats, based on the theory that saturated fat intake spikes cholesterol levels, and high cholesterol leads to heart disease. According to this theory, elevated cholesterol levels in the arteries leads to *atherosclerosis*, or a blockage that cuts off blood supply to the heart and other organs and tissues. Naturally, this led to the belief that heart disease is the result of a diet high in saturated fats.

For decades, the medical profession has urged us all to avoid eating too much saturated fat and cholesterol-containing foods. Cholesterol-lowering drugs, known as *statins*, continue to be the most widely prescribed class of medications in the United States. Studies show, however, that statin drugs offer no preventive benefits that protect against heart attacks, and therefore should only be prescribed to people who have already experienced a heart attack in order to stop another one. And even then, the research has also shown that there are far more effective approaches for preventing a recurrence of heart attack than statins provide, starting with a healthy diet and lifestyle. In spite of this evidence, statins are still the most profitable drugs in the United States, with many doctors even calling for their issuance to pre-teens and teenagers to prevent heart disease.

But is cholesterol truly the villain in the story of heart disease?

In a word, no!

In fact, you would not be alive were it not for cholesterol. The proof of that statement is provided by your body itself, which manufactures between 80 to 90 percent of all the cholesterol in your system, primarily in your liver. It has to, because cholesterol is essential for many of the functions that keep you alive and healthy. It is a major structural component of every cell in your body and plays an especially important role in maintaining the integrity of the cell membrane, which encloses and protects the cells themselves. Cholesterol is used by the body to manufacture various hormones, including estrogen and testosterone, as well as vitamin D from the sun (vitamin D acts far more like a hormone than it does a vitamin). Your body also needs cholesterol to produce fat-soluble vitamins, as well as the bile salts that your body requires for the proper absorption of fats.

Cholesterol also acts as a natural anti-inflammatory agent. When inflammation is present in the body, cholesterol levels automatically rise as the body attempts to cope with it. This is especially true when unhealthy, acidifying, and inflammation-causing foods and beverages are consumed.

While it is true that certain foods high in saturated fats, such as dairy products, eggs, meats, and yes, coconuts, also contain cholesterol, the diet of the average American today only contains between 250 to 350 mg of cholesterol. In comparison, each and every day, your liver produces around 1000 mg of cholesterol. Moreover, studies have shown that when people eliminate or restrict their intake of cholesterol-rich foods, liver production of cholesterol increases by as much as an additional 500 mg. Given that the human body is designed to keep itself alive through a continuous repair and adjustment process known as *homeostasis*, why would it produce so much cholesterol if cholesterol poses a threat to its health?

Proponents of the high cholesterol theory of heart disease answer this question by claiming that there are both "good" and "bad" kinds of cholesterol. Good cholesterol is known as high-density lipoprotein (HDL), and bad cholesterol is known as low-density lipoprotein (LDL). But the distinction between HDL and LDL cholesterol is not as clear cut as it is commonly believed to be. In actuality, both forms of cholesterol are the same. What is different is the roles that HDL and LDL play in your body. HDL acts to return cholesterol from your body's tissues back to the liver, while LDL acts to transport cholesterol from the liver out to the rest of your body.

To better understand this point, imagine two lines of workers in a factory, carrying materials to and from a machine shop. Would you characterize the workers who returned the materials to the machine shop as any better than the workers who carried the materials away from the shop if those duties were precisely what the workers were hired to do? No, of course you wouldn't.

Similarly, it makes just as little sense to characterize LDL as "bad cholesterol" when it is simply carrying out the tasks it was designed to do, just as so-called "good" HDL is doing. But LDL is still branded as bad because of its link to heart disease when it becomes oxidized, or "rusts." But there is a big difference between LDL cholesterol by itself and oxidized LDL cholesterol. Only oxidized LDL cholesterol has been shown to be a risk factor for heart disease. This is a very important point to understand. In Chapter 4, you will learn how and why the inclusion of coconuts and coconut oil in your diet can prevent cholesterol from becoming oxidized.

Given the "bad rap" that cholesterol has received, you might be asking yourself how it came to be so demonized in the first place. To answer that a bit of history is in order. The high cholesterol theory of heart disease originated in the early 20th century. In December 1912, the American physician James B. Herrick, MD published what is considered to be the most influential medical article to first focus doctors on blockages of the coronary artery. Entitled "Clinical Features of Sudden Obstruction of the Coronary Arteries," its appearance in the *Journal of the American Medical Association* (JAMA) is credited with aligning the various factions of doctors and their respective theories about the cause of heart disease. Not coincidentally, it was around this same time that the modern day field of cardiology began to be formed and defined.

A year later, halfway around the world, a Russian pathologist, Nikolai N. Anitschkow, laid the foundation for the demonization of cholesterol through his experiments with animals. Specifically, he fed purified cholesterol dissolved in sunflower oil to rabbits. Over time, the rabbits went on to develop lesions in their arteries that closely resembled the lesions that occur in humans when atherosclerosis develops. Based on his findings, Anitschkow concluded that cholesterol was the cause of atherosclerosis. Unfortunately, he, like many researchers before and after him, mistook a correlation for a cause.

Moreover, Anitschkow never seems to have considered the fact that rabbits are herbivores, and therefore do not obtain cholesterol from their natural diet. Or perhaps he chose to ignore this fact, given that his research stemmed from earlier experiments at the medical school where he received his training showing that rabbits fed a diet high in protein quickly began to age at an accelerated pace. In young rabbits, such a diet, which consisted of large amounts of eggs, milk, and meat (again, not what rabbits normally eat) led to significant declines in adrenal and liver function, while in adult rabbits it too led to atherosclerosis.

Follow-up studies by other researchers involving dogs and rats failed to duplicate Anitschkow's findings. This is not surprising, since these animals are meat-eaters and normally obtain cholesterol in their diets. And it was later discovered that it was not the elevated cholesterol Anitschkow's rabbits were fed that caused their atherosclerosis, but rather depressed thyroid function triggered by the cholesterol due to the fact that rabbits are not designed by nature to eat high cholesterol foods. But by then it was too late. Despite the fact that Anitschkow apparently glossed over the fact that the diets he forced on the rabbits were entirely unnatural to their makeup, the link between cholesterol and atherosclerosis (and therefore, heart disease) had already taken hold.

But it was not until the 1950s on into the present that cholesterol truly began to be demonized, largely due to the work and research of Ancel Keys, PhD. Keys was the founding director of the Laboratory of Physiological Hygiene at the University of Minnesota and also served with the United States Quartermaster Army Corps. While there, he contributed to the war effort during World War II by developing the K-rations that are named after him, enabling United States troops to sustain themselves for up to two weeks in the field eating the portable and nonperishable food items the K-rations contained. After World War II, he was alarmed by research showing that

American business executives were experiencing high rates of heart disease, whereas in postwar Europe, rates of heart disease had plummeted.

Keys suspected that the sharp reduction in food supplies following the war explained the drop in European heart disease rates, and that the rich diet of the American executives was responsible for their poor health. To prove his hypothesis, he conducted what became known as the Seven Countries Study, which focused on the diets of populations in Finland, Greece, Japan, Italy, Netherlands, Yugoslavia, and the United States. Based on his findings, Keys claimed that cholesterol levels was strongly related to heart disease mortality, both at the individual level and among general populations.

In addition to Keys' Seven Countries Study, only six other major long-term clinical trials were ever conducted that support the high cholesterol/ blocked artery model of heart disease. They are the *Air Force*/Texas Coronary Atherosclerosis Prevention Study; the Anglo Scandinavian Cardiac Outcomes Trial; the Helsinki Heart Study; the Lipid Research Clinics Coronary Primary Prevention Trial; the West of Scotland Coronary Prevention Study Group; and World Health Organization (WHO) Cooperative Trial.

In each of these trials, statin drugs were administered to test subjects to lower serum cholesterol levels. The results of the studies are worth noting. First of all, there was no statistical difference in the rate of death caused by heart disease between test subjects who received statins and the control groups. Far more alarming, in two of the clinical trials (Helsinki and WHO) there was a significantly higher rate of cancer deaths—18 to 24 percent— among test subjects given statin drugs compared to the control group. Despite these occurrences, lowering cholesterol levels through the use of statin drugs continues to be advised by both the pharmaceutical industry and major medical associations, such as the American Medical Association (AMA), the American Heart Association, and the National Lung and Blood Institute.

Although critics at the time claimed that Keys buried the findings of fifteen other countries that contradicted the results of his study, Keys remained adamant that dietary saturated fats caused elevated cholesterol levels, which in turn caused heart disease and was the culprit behind heart attacks being the number one cause of death in the U.S.

Yet, in 1957, the American Heart Association (AHA), disputed this view, stating at the time that "the evidence that dietary fat correlates with heart disease *does not stand up* to critical examination." It was not until 1961 that the AHA reversed its position and joined forces with Keys after he became an AHA committee member. It was this committee that issued a report, entitled "Dietary fat and its relation to heart attacks and strokes," which stated that a low-fat diet was necessary to avoid the risk of heart disease.

Following the report's publication, AHA spokespersons took to the media to warn the American public about the dangers of saturated fat food sources in relation to heart disease. The government quickly followed suit, issuing federal guidelines recommending that a low-fat diet be followed in order to prevent heart disease and recommending monounsaturated fats and PUFAs as the only healthy fats to eat. After that, it was not long before the high cholesterol theory of heart disease and the importance of a low-fat diet both began to be accepted as facts throughout many other countries around the world. The belief that this is so still persists today.

Now that you understand the history and premise of this model for heart disease, let's see how well it actually holds up. The short answer is: Not well at all. But don't take my word for it. Instead, let's look at statements by Keys himself. Despite being the primary proponent of the cholesterol theory of heart disease, even Keys came to admit that cholesterol in and of itself was hardly the culprit he once claimed it was. In 1987 he was quoted in the *New York Times,* saying, "I've come to think that cholesterol is not as important as we used to think it was. Let's reduce cholesterol by reasonable means, but let's not get too excited about it." A few years later, in 1991, Keys wrote a letter to *New England Journal of Medicine,* explaining, "There's no connection whatsoever between cholesterol in food and cholesterol in blood and we've known that all along. Cholesterol in the diet doesn't matter unless you happen to be a chicken or a rabbit."

The fact that Keys late in his life admitted that he was wrong about cholesterol is significant, yet his admissions have not received the same amount of publicity and support that his earlier, anti-cholesterol statements have. Nonetheless, a growing body of evidence continues to prove that Keys' mid-20th century research is wrong. Consider, for example, the following facts:

- The standard American diet lacks the nutrition to maintain healthy HDL.

- Numerous studies show that people with high cholesterol live the longest.

- In subjects seventy and older, those *not* receiving cholesterol-lowering statin drugs lived the longest.

- In a Canadian study of 5,000 men tracked over twelve years, cholesterol was *not* associated with heart disease.

- On average, men suffer heart attacks at a rate 3 to 5 times greater than that of women, yet women typically have higher cholesterol levels than men.

- The incidence of heart attacks is spread pretty evenly across the entire spectrum of cholesterol levels.

- Half of the people who are hospitalized with heart attacks have normal cholesterol levels.

- Numerous studies, including the famed Framingham Heart Study and the World Health Organization's MONICA Study, have found minimal links between cholesterol levels and heart disease, and what correlation does exist typically disappears by age fifty.

- The Framingham Heart Study has found that low LDL cholesterol levels may increase the risk of the future development of cancer.

- In a study of 120 subjects with second heart attacks, the number with low cholesterol vs. those with high cholesterol was almost identical.

- Low cholesterol levels have also been linked to impaired immune function, and connected to the development of neurological disorders, including Parkinson's and Alzheimer's disease. (This is not surprising, since the human brain requires large amounts of cholesterol, as well as saturated fats, to maintain its health and function properly.)

Given all of the above, you can understand why I view the high cholesterol theory of heart disease as being highly flawed. Nor am I alone. More and more doctors are coming to recognize that this theory simply cannot account for how and why heart disease develops.

Among them, it may surprise you to know, is George V. Mann, ScD, MD, professor of Biochemistry at Vanderbilt School of Medicine, and the co-director of the Framingham Heart Study, who says, "Saturated fat and cholesterol in the diet are not the cause of coronary heart disease. That myth is the greatest 'scientific' deception of the century, and perhaps any century."

Most recently, Dr. Mann's views were bolstered by an opinion piece published in the *British Journal of Sports Medicine* entitled "Saturated fat does not clog the arteries: coronary heart disease is a chronic inflammatory condition, the risk of which can be effectively reduced from healthy lifestyle interventions." It was written by three cardiologists and world-renowned experts in heart disease: Aseem Malhotra, Rita Redberg, and Pascal Meier.

In the article, the authors asserted that, "Despite popular belief among doctors and the public, the conceptual model of dietary saturated fat clogging a pipe [artery] is just plain wrong. A landmark systematic review and meta-analysis of observational studies showed no association between saturated fat consumption and (1) all-cause mortality, (2) coronary heart disease (CHD), (3) CHD mortality, (4) ischemic stroke or (5) type 2 diabetes in healthy adults. Similarly in the secondary prevention of CHD there is no benefit from reduced fat, including saturated fat, on myocardial infarction, cardiovascular or all-cause mortality. It is instructive to note that in an angiographic study of postmenopausal women with CHD, greater intake of saturated fat was associated with less progression of atherosclerosis whereas carbohydrate and polyunsaturated fat intake were associated with greater progression."

Drs. Mahlotra, Redberg, and Meier point out that the real culprit in heart disease, stroke, and other diseases is chronic inflammation. As you will discover in Chapter 4, the saturated fats found in coconuts and coconut oil provide powerful anti-inflammatory benefits, which is one of the reasons why regularly consuming coconuts and its oil can improve heart health.

Unsaturated Fats: The Good and the Not So Good

While a growing body of scientific evidence confirms the fact that saturated fats are actually essential for good overall health and not unhealthy as they were once thought to be, this does not mean unsaturated fats are unhealthy as well. The simple truth is that all fats that naturally occur in foods are good for us, whereas trans fats, which are manmade, are most definitely not.

The problem with unsaturated fats lies in how prevalent they have become in our diet today. The balance between the omega-3 and omega-6 oils in unsaturated fats has increasingly been disrupted. Omega-3 and omega-6 oils are both essential fatty acids (EFAs), meaning that they are vitally important for good health. EFAs make up part of the body's cell membranes and are particularly concentrated in the adrenal glands, brain cells, eyes, nerve cells, and the sex glands. Without enough EFAs, your body cannot adequately produce enough energy, regulate hormone production and proper nerve function, maintain brain health, and maintain the proper functioning of its overall musculoskeletal system. Since EFAs are not produced by your body, they must be obtained either through the foods you eat or as omega oil supplements.

Too Much of a Good Thing

For much of human history, the balance between omega-3 and omega-6 fatty acids in our diets was approximately 1:1. This healthy ratio range is what nature intended. But by the mid-1800s, around the end of the Industrial Revolution, omega-6 acids became more prevalent in the American diet than omega-3s. This change in ratio corresponded with the dawn of the modern vegetable oil industry and was further accelerated by a shift in livestock feeding methods from grass-feeding to a cereal grain-based diet. This shift occurred despite the fact that livestock do not naturally prefer cereal grains.

By the 1930s, research shows that the 1:1 ratio between omega-3s and omega-6s in the human diet had already changed to more than 1:8 in favor of omega-6 fatty acids. Today, that ratio has been skewed even more, to as much as 1:15, and for some people it's as much as 1:25. In fact, researchers have established that at least 9 percent of the total amount of calories consumed by the average American today come from polyunsaturated fats high in omega-6 fatty acids. What is most alarming about this finding is that research has also established that omega-6s begin to create toxicity in our bodies when they exceed 4 percent of our total daily caloric intake.

One of the main reasons why we are consuming far too much omega-6 oils is because of how widespread the use of vegetable oils has become. These oils, which are polyunsaturated, include canola oil, corn oil, soybean oil, sunflower oil, and many others. Margarine and vegetable shortening are other commonly used food ingredients that are very high in omega-6 fatty acids. Margarine is also primarily composed of unhealthy trans fats.

Not only are these oils commonly used at home as a cheaper alternative to healthier oils, such as flaxseed and olive oil (both oils that are high in omega-3 fatty acids), they are staple ingredients in many canned and packaged foods, including many packaged products that are considered to be "health foods." Moreover, due to their lower cost, these types of oils are used in many restaurants and other dining establishments across the United States. As a result, the excessive consumption of omega-6 fatty acids has become extremely hard to avoid until you become aware of the problem and then take the necessary actions to correct it. Check the labels of canned and packaged foods when you go shopping, and try to limit your use of vegetable oil and other unsaturated oils in your cooking and baking.

Chronic Inflammation and Oxidation

The biggest health threats posed by excess unsaturated fat consumption are their tendency to cause chronic inflammation and oxidation within the tissues and organs of the body. The body's inflammatory response is one of the ways in which it acts to protect and heal itself from injury, trauma, and infection. Diseases that ends in "-itis" are caused by chronic inflammation in the body, particularly within the organ the disease corresponds to. Oxidation, if excessive, can cause tissues and organs to "rust," in the same way that an apple, when cut and exposed to air, rapidly begins to turn brown as it comes in contact with the oxygen the air contains.

Oxidation occurs in the body when atoms lose an electron. These missing electrons are replaced by substances known as free radicals. Free radical damage is a major health risk, which is why nutritional supplements and foods rich in antioxidants are so often recommended by nutritionally-oriented physicians. Antioxidants "quench" free radicals, helping to prevent damage to the body's cells, tissues, and organs caused by oxidative stress. But what does this have to do with unsaturated fats, you might ask?

Quite a lot.

To understand why, let's return to the double carbon bonds found in unsaturated oils, especially PUFAs. Double carbon bonds act as "weak links" in the carbon chains that are found in all fats. The weakness in this case being that double carbon bonds are highly susceptible to oxidation, which in turn triggers and further exacerbates chronic inflammation in the body.

But it is not the omega-3s found in these types of fats that are causing the problem of inflammation. Omega-3 fatty acids actually act as natural anti-inflammatory substances in the body once they are consumed. This is why fish and fish oil supplements, both of which are rich in omega-3s, are now so often recommended by physicians to help protect against heart disease, as well as arthritis and many other inflammatory disease conditions.

Omega-6 fatty acids, on the other hand, have a pro-inflammatory effect in the body.

Omega-6 fatty acids are so prominent in the typical American diet that instead of being beneficial to our health, they are one of the primary dietary factors wrecking havoc on it. Excess consumption of omega-6s found in PUFAs are known to cause or worsen a wide range of serious chronic and degenerative diseases. These include autoimmune conditions, cancer, cardiovascular disease, diabetes, gastrointestinal conditions, psychiatric disorders, respiratory conditions such as asthma and bronchitis, and even vision problems, including macular degeneration.

The widespread prevalence of omega-6 fatty acids in our diet is also playing a major causative role in our nation's obesity epidemic. This fact has been

Are You Eating Wood Varnish?

Here's an interesting fact not many people know about: A number of common polyunsaturated oils are often used to varnish wood, precisely because of their high rate of oxidation. When these oils oxidize, they form a polymer type film on the wood, which becomes the varnish. (Polymers are large molecules made up of chains or rings of smaller molecular units.) Now that you know this, ask yourself if you think it wise to consume a lot of oils that act as wood varnish.

demonstrated by a number of research studies, such as one which found that levels of PUFA fats stored in body fat have increased by 136 percent in correlation with an increase in dietary linoleic acid, a type of omega-6. Based on the above facts, you can clearly see why unsaturated fats, especially polyunsaturated fats high in omega-6s, are hardly the healthy fat choices that we for far too long have been told they are.

THE REALITY: SATURATED FATS ARE GOOD FOR YOU

Imagine a food substance that, for many centuries, had been a naturally-occurring staple of the diets of peoples all around the world, and during all that time there had never been any indication that this ingredient was harmful. Then, as a result of a series of flawed yet widely publicized studies, suddenly this substance was claimed to be unhealthy and something that should be avoided. And then imagine, even after the studies' claims were shown to be erroneous, with, decades later, still no tangible evidence to support them, physicians, government health agencies, and other health authorities still continued to warn the public that the substance was a health risk. This is precisely what has happened to naturally occurring saturated fats, which are found in foods derived from both animals and certain plants.

Earlier in this chapter, I explained that saturated fats were first demonized by a series of studies that linked them to high cholesterol, based on the assumption that heart disease is caused by high cholesterol. The claim that high cholesterol leads to heart disease is, in fact, flawed, and even the primary proponent of this theory, Ancel Keys, eventually came to admit that cholesterol in the diet actually did not matter. But even today his admission remains largely ignored by the medical profession, which for the most part continues to recommend a low-fat diet. Meanwhile, the pharmaceutical industry continues to influence doctors to push cholesterol-lowering statin drugs, all of which are known to carry the risk of serious side effects.

The truth is a certain amount of both saturated fats and dietary cholesterol are essential to good health and need to be included in your diet. Contrary to popular opinion, saturated fat is important for the health of your heart and overall cardiovascular system. The heart itself is surrounded by a protective layer of saturated fat, which helps regulate cholesterol levels, supplies the heart with energy, and prevents plaque buildup in the arteries. Adequate amounts of saturated fats in the diet have also been shown to reduce levels of lipoprotein(a), a substance which can significantly increase the risk of heart attack, stroke, and other types of heart disease. In addition, dietary saturated fats help to increase levels of HDL, or "good" cholesterol, further reducing the risk of heart disease.

Dietary saturated fats also help to prevent unhealthy weight gain and act as effective weight loss foods. Eating food rich in saturated fats results in quicker satiety—feeling full—so that people are less apt to overeat at meals. Saturated fats are slowly absorbed by the body, so the experience of satiety lasts longer than it does from eating low-fat foods, making it easier to go longer between meals without feeling hungry.

Certain saturated fats, especially those found in coconuts and coconut oil, have been shown to help reduce stored abdominal fat, which is one of the hardest fats to lose and a major risk factor for heart disease, diabetes, and hormonal imbalances. When foods rich in saturated foods are consumed in place of high carbohydrate foods, rather than being stored in the body, the fats stimulate stored body fat to be released and used for energy, thus improving a person's ability to lose weight. This fact is backed by a number of studies, all of which have found that dieters who consume the greatest percentage of saturated fats tend to lose the most weight and are able to most successfully keep it off.

Saturated fats also provide countless health benefits beyond cardiovascular and dietary health. Our bodies are designed from birth to thrive on saturated fats—the total fat content of human breast milk is approximately 50 percent. The human brain, which does not fully develop until about age twelve, requires and produces large amounts of saturated fatty acids as it matures.

Saturated fats and cholesterol make up a large part of our body's myelin sheaths, which coat and protect nerve fibers in the brain to ensure that nerve cells can properly transmit information and assist in other complex brain processes. Overall, over 50 percent of the brain is composed of fats and cholesterol. Saturated fats serve as a vitally important raw material, which the brain requires to maintain its health, grow, and regenerate.

Dietary saturated fats help the body absorb and better utilize minerals and other nutrients. The fats themselves are rich sources of the essential fat-soluble vitamins A, D, E, and K. Among these vitamins' many health benefits are protecting the health of the eyes and skin by acting as a lubricant to prevent both eyes and skin from becoming too dry.

Saturated fats are the building blocks for the body's cell membranes. At least 50 percent of the cell membranes are composed of saturated fatty acids. Without saturated fats, cell membranes would be unable to maintain their shape and structural integrity, which is necessary for oxygen and nutrients to pass into cells, and for cellular wastes to pass out from them.

Without sufficient levels of saturated fats, the ability of the immune system's white blood cells to recognize and eliminate infectious agents, such as harmful bacteria, viruses, and other microbes, can be significantly diminished. Dietary saturated fats also help to protect against harmful microorganisms taking hold within the gastrointestinal tract.

Saturated fats are also beneficial for lung and liver health. They help to protect the liver from harm caused by toxins, including the toxic side effects caused by alcohol and pharmaceutical drugs, especially nonsteroidal anti-inflammatory drugs (NSAIDs), such as acetaminophen (Tylenol), ibuprofen (Motrin), and even aspirin, all of which can impair liver function over time if they are regularly consumed. In order for your lungs to function properly, their airspaces must be coated with a thin, protective layer known as lung surfactant, which is composed entirely of saturated fat. A lack of saturated fats in the diet can result in deterioration of this protective coating, leading to difficulties breathing and various types of lung disease.

Given all of the above benefits of saturated fats, you can see why making saturated fats a part of your daily diet is so important. Now let's examine the particular type of saturated fat found in coconuts and coconut oil, including the healthy advantages it provides compared to other saturated fats.

THE COCONUT MCFA DIFFERENCE

There is one major difference between the saturated fat content of coconuts, as well as coconut oil, and the saturated fats derived from other food sources. The difference is that the fats in coconut are medium-chain fatty acid (MCFAs), also known as a medium-chain triglycerides (MCTs). By contrast, the saturated and unsaturated fats in other foods (both animal and plant foods) are made up of long-chain fatty acids (LCFAs). Compared to LCFAs, MCFAs are more easily digested than other fats. More importantly, unlike LCFAs, which get stored in your body's other cells, tissues, and organs, MCFAs are stored in the liver, where they are quickly metabolized and converted into a readily available source of energy.

Nearly half—45 percent—of the fat in coconut oil is in the form of lauric acid, a substance your body converts into monolaurin. Monolaurin is the same compound found in breast milk that is used to boost the immune system of newborn babies. Research has also shown that monolaurin helps protect the health of the brain and plays an important role in maintaining the health of your body's bones. Moreover, lauric acid stimulates the conversion of LDL cholesterol into pregnenolone, a substance the body requires to produce and maintain its supply of hormones, thereby changing a potentially harmful substance into something that has positive health benefits.

In addition to lauric acid, the fat from coconuts also contain capric and caprylic acids. Together, these three fatty acids provide a variety of important health benefits. They act as an excellent source of energy in the body because coconut's three fatty acids only require a three-step conversion process by the body to be digested and made available as a fuel source, unlike other fatty acids from both saturated and unsaturated foods, which have to undergo a 26-step process before they are fully digested and can be used by the body. MCFAs are also much easier to digest compared to LCFAs, are not as readily stored by the body as fat, and are smaller in size, making it easier for them to pass through cell membranes to immediately begin providing energy.

In addition to these superior benefits of the MCFAs contained in coconuts, research shows that MCFAs from coconuts:

- Regulate blood sugar levels and protect against insulin resistance, thereby helping to prevent type 2 diabetes.

- Regulate cholesterol levels by both increasing healthy HDL cholesterol and lowering unhealthy LDL levels.

- Aid in weight loss by curbing appetite, boosting metabolism, improving the body's ability to burn calories, and reducing abdominal fat.

- Act as antioxidants, helping to prevent and reduce free radical damage that can lead to disease and premature aging.

- Aid the immune system by targeting and eliminating harmful bacteria, viruses, and fungi.

- Help regulate blood pressure levels and prevent hypertension, or high blood pressure.

- Reduce inflammation.

- Aid in the absorption of nutrients from food while also protecting the health of the gastrointestinal tract.

- Protect against gum disease.

- Boost energy levels in the body.

- Protect the brain by aiding in the liver's production of ketones, substances that the brain breaks down into energy when other energy sources, such as glucose, are low. Research shows that the brains of people suffering from dementia and Alzheimer's disease have lost the ability to create insulin, suggesting that ketones produced from consuming coconuts and coconut oil might help compensate for this lost ability by supplying an alternate source of energy to help repair brain function.

In addition, because MCFAs in coconuts and coconut oil do not oxidize as rapidly as the LCFAs found in monounsaturated and polyunsaturated oils, coconut oil is a healthier choice for cooking. Heat from cooking can destroy the beneficial fats in most oils. This is particularly true of vegetable oils, including olive oil, which are most susceptible to high temperatures that can cause the fats they contain to become damaged and turn inflammatory and even carcinogenic. Coconut oil has a much higher heat, or smoking, point and therefore is much better able to withstand higher temperatures without its fats becoming damaged and dangerous to your health. In addition, cooking with coconut oil can also enhance the flavor and texture of foods cooked in it.

CONCLUSION

Now that you have read this chapter, it is my hope that you have a better understanding of why fats, including saturated and unsaturated fats, are essential for your good health and a necessary component of your daily dietary intake. By maintaining a healthy diet that includes saturated fats and a proper balance of omega-3 and omega-6 fatty acids found in unsaturated fats, you will go a long way towards preventing the scourges of chronic inflammation as well as helping to protect yourself against many of today's chronic, degenerative diseases. This includes our nation's number one killer—heart disease. In the next chapter you will discover the important ways in which adding coconut and coconut oil to your diet can help keep your heart protected and healthy.

4.

Coconuts
and Your Heart

Your heart is one of the most important organs in your body, perhaps the most important, even more so than your brain. And in today's world it is under constant assault due to a combination of chronic stress, poor diet and nutrition, and the onslaught of environmental toxins found in our air, water, soil, and food.

Since the beginning of the 20th century, heart disease in the United States has been our nation's number one killer. Nor is it likely to give up that position any time soon. Consider these grim statistics:

- More than 2,200 Americans die of heart disease each and every day. That's an average of one death every 39 seconds.

- An average of 150,000 Americans who die of heart disease each year are younger than 65 years of age, while 33 percent of all deaths caused by heart disease occur before the age of 75 years, which is well below the average life expectancy of 77.9 years.

- Coronary heart disease causes one of every six deaths in the United States, each year, while one out of every 18 deaths is caused by stroke.

- Nearly 634,000 Americans die of heart disease each year.

- Each year, an estimated 785,000 Americans have a heart attack, and 470,000 more have a repeat attack.

- Approximately 195,000 Americans experience a silent (unnoticed or undiagnosed) first myocardial infarction each year.

- Approximately every 25 seconds, an American will have a coronary event, and approximately every minute, someone will die of one.

Once mistakenly thought to primarily affect men, approximately 50 percent of all deaths caused by heart disease in the U.S. each year occur among women, accounting for more than six times the number of deaths caused by breast cancer. Though mortality rates caused by heart disease have started to decline over the past decade, the overall toll continues to rise, both in terms of impaired health and financial cost. More than 1,100,000 inpatient angioplasty procedures are performed in the U.S. each year, along with 416,000 inpatient bypass procedures, more than 1,000,000 inpatient diagnostic cardiac catheterizations, 116,000 inpatient implantable defibrillator procedures, and 397,000 pacemaker procedures.

Annually, heart disease in the United States accounts for direct and indirect costs of more than $190.3 billion, and predictions are that these costs will increase by a minimum of 200 percent over the next 20 years. And that does not include the additional tens of billions of dollars that are spent each year to manage risk factors associated with heart disease, such as the $19 billion spent annually on statin drugs to treat elevated cholesterol levels.

Certainly there would be no reason to object to these staggering financial costs if the procedures and medications used to treat heart disease truly did their job. Unfortunately, all too often they do not. Studies show that far too common surgical procedures, such as angioplasty and bypass, are of questionable value in terms of long-term health outcomes and can even make patient's conditions worse due to doctor error. Additional studies are also now calling into question the use of statin drugs, especially as a preventive measure for heart attack.

Moreover, researchers from McMaster University in Ontario, Canada, recently discovered that nearly half of all patients who are prescribed cholesterol-lowering statin drugs get no benefit from them due to high blood levels of a protein called resistin. Resistin, which is secreted by fat tissue, causes the formation of LDL cholesterol, thus counteracting any positive effects statin drugs may have.

Overall, although the overall incidence of death caused by heart disease is at last beginning to show signs of decline, the cost involved in treating and preventing it continues to rise at an alarming rate, and many patients continue to suffer declining quality of life issues due to the procedures and medications they receive. Surely there has to be a better way to treat and prevent our nation's number one health scourge.

While the search for such solutions continues, one of the things you can do right now to protect your heart is to include coconuts and coconut oil as part of your daily diet. This fact has been confirmed by studies of people who traditionally follow a diet high in coconuts and coconut milk and water, and who cook with coconut oil, including Pacific Islanders and Sri Lanka. Research has shown that people in these regions who follow such diets and who use coconut oil for their food preparations have a very low incidence of heart disease. But when these peoples move away from coconut-rich diets to adopt Western diets, within one or two generations, their incidence of heart disease mirrors the same rate as that here in the States.

To understand why this is so, let's first take a closer look at the magnificent organ that your heart is and explore a bit more what causes heart disease.

MEET YOUR HEART

The human heart is the very first organ to form in the developing fetus. It begins to take shape only 18 days after conception, and by day 22 it is already starting to beat and pulse. As it develops, it forms specialized muscles comprised of not just the four heart chambers (the upper left and right chambers, called atria, and the lower left and right chambers, known as the ventricles) but also the muscle cells of the veins and arteries, as well as the tissues that make up the valves and other aspects of the heart. This complex, interrelated network is known as the cardiovascular system, also known as the circulatory system.

In addition to the heart itself, four main types of blood vessels make up your body's cardiovascular system: arteries, veins, capillaries, and sinuoids. All of them are shaped like hollow tubes, with both the arteries and veins, when they are healthy also having a high degree of elasticity so that blood can flow freely through them. Combined, if all of your body's blood vessels were stretched out end to end they would be about 60,000 miles long. That's more than twice the circumference of the earth. This astonishing fact is even more amazing when you realize that your heart moves the approximately six quarts (5.6 liters) of blood that are contained in the adult human body through this entire network an average of three times every minute of your life (once every 20 seconds).

Complex as your cardiovascular system is in general, your heart is even more so. In fact, it is the most complex of all your body's organs. Though most people think of the heart simply as an organ that pumps blood, it does far more than that. It also acts like an endocrine gland, producing its own hormones, and has a rich neural tissue, comparable to the neural tissue of your brain. Perhaps this is why, throughout civilizations of the distant past, the heart was regarded as the seat of both intelligence and intuition.

In ancient Greece, the heart was believed to be the seat of the soul, or spirit, while the ancient Chinese recognized the heart as the center for happiness. The Greeks were also the first to associate the heart with love.

In ancient Egypt, the heart was regarded as the source of both intelligence and emotions. In fact, prior to the process of mummification, the Egyptians cut out the brain from the body and disposed of it because it was deemed unimportant, while the heart was protected so that it could guide the deceased into the afterlife.

Research has established that the heart is the greatest source of electro-magnetic energy in the body. Its electrical field is 60 times greater than that of the brain, while the heart's magnetic field is 5,000 times stronger than the brain's. This cardio-electromagnetic field has been measured and extends between eight to ten feet from your body. Researchers now theorize that this field acts as a "carrier wave" of and for information, providing a global syn-chronizing signal for the entire human body.

Here are some other amazing facts about your heart:

- On average the adult human heart only weighs between 8 and 10 ounces in women and men respectively, and is about the size of a fist (approximately 3.5 by 5 inches).

- Although many people believe the heart is located on the left side of their chest, in reality it is located in the center of the chest, between both lungs. Your left lung is smaller than your right lung, however, so that your heart can fit within your chest cavity.

- Your heart is almost entirely composed of muscle and the amount of work that it performs in a single hour is enough to lift a small car weighing approximately 3,000 pounds one foot off the ground.

- The heart beats an average of 103,000 times per day every day of your life. That equates to approximately 3,600,000 times a year, and 2.5 billion times over a 70-year-long lifespan.

- The heartbeat in women is faster than it is in men.

- The average amount of blood pumped per heartbeat when you are at rest is 2.5 ounces. Over the course of 24 hours that is nearly 2,000 gallons (approximately 20,000 pounds) of blood that your heart has moved.

- The pressure created in your heart during a single heartbeat is enough to squirt blood a distance of nearly 30 feet.

- The sound of your heartbeat is caused by closing of the valves that sepa-rate the atria from the ventricle (atrioventricular valves).

- Electrical impulses in the heart muscle (myocardium) are what cause your heart to beat.

- Laughing is very beneficial for your heart and can improve blood flow for up to 45 minutes after you stop laughing.

- Your heart replaces your body's entire store of ATP (*adenosine triphosphate*, your body's main source of energy) 8,640 times per day, or once every 10 seconds.

COCONUTS CAN HELP KEEP YOUR HEART HEALTHY

There are a number of components that act together to maintain the health of the heart and the overall cardiovascular system. When the "rhythmic" interplay between these components functions as nature intended, all is well, but when this rhythm becomes unbalanced, heart disease follows. Adding coconuts and coconut milk and oil to your diet can be beneficial to the chemical, electrical, and structural components.

Chemical

The mix of hormones and chemicals coursing through heart muscles is nothing short of amazing. But when their balance is disrupted this results in a cascade of metabolic chaos for heart muscle cells, in particular, and for heart muscle tissues (the myocardium), in general.

Electrical

In order for cells, including heart cells, to remain healthy electrolyte balance is critical. Electrolytes are minerals, such as potassium, calcium, sodium, magnesium, and chloride that help maintain proper fluid levels in the body and regulate heart function, as well as the functioning of all other muscles in the body. When electrolytes become imbalanced, the critical process of creating energy slows down inside cells. This, in turn, causes cell membranes to lose their integrity, which is maintained by the membranes' electrical charge.

As cell membrane integrity is lost, the membrane becomes increasingly permeable, enabling substances that do not belong inside the cells to pass into the cell, while at the same time interfering with the passage of vital compounds, as well as waste matter, out of the cell. Soon, this disrupts what is known as the "sodium/potassium pump." This, in turn, disrupts the cellular channel that controls levels of both sodium and calcium, allowing too much sodium and calcium to enter the cell and the mitochondria (your cells' "energy factories"). Once inside the mitochondria, calcium starts to disrupt critical enzyme pathways, causing cells to die.

Structural

Cellular structural integrity also plays a critical role in optimal cell function, including that of heart muscle cells. Fatty acid compounds known as phospholipids compose cell membranes. When the structure of the phospholipids begins to break down, cell membranes become "leaky." As this process continues, abnormalities within the phospholipids also progress, altering other structural compounds of the cell membranes.

All of the major types of heart disease occur, in part, because of a breakdown in one or more of the components.

Coconuts, coconut milk, coconut water, and coconut oil can all help to prevent such breakdowns. First, they help to protect and maintain the heart's electrical component because they are rich in electrolyte minerals, especially potassium, sodium, calcium, magnesium, and phosphorus. Coconuts and their milk, water, and oil contain nearly twice as much potassium per serving (600 mg per cup) than bananas (360 mg per cup), which are famous for being a potassium-rich food. Research has found that potassium is particularly important for the proper regulation of the cellular functioning of heart muscle cells.

Coconuts, coconut milk and water, and coconut oil also provide a healthy amount of sodium (salt), which, like cholesterol, has been demonized as a health threat. The truth of the matter, however, is that a certain amount of sodium in the diet is essential for optimal health, including the health of the heart and cardiovascular system. Without enough sodium, your body cannot maintain proper fluid balance. In addition, the most common electrolyte disorder among Americans today is a condition known as *hyponatremia,* a potentially fatal condition characterized by sodium levels in the body that are too low.

Your heart's electrical system also requires calcium, magnesium, and phosphorus in order to function properly. All three of these minerals are found in coconuts, coconut milk and water, and coconut oil.

The fatty acids found in coconuts and its milk, water, and oil can also help to maintain the structural integrity of heart cells by supplying the phospholipids necessary for cellular membranes to stay healthy and intact. The structural integrity of heart cells is vitally important. Without such integrity, oxygen and vital nutrients that the cells require to produce energy cannot efficiently pass into the cells from the bloodstream. In addition, as cell structures become impaired, cellular waste matter can become trapped inside heart cells, further impairing their functioning, including the production of energy that your heart requires.

Coconuts and their milk, water, and oil also help to produce and naturally balance hormones in the body because of the cholesterol, fatty acids (especially lauric acid), and various amino acids, B vitamins, and minerals that are found in coconuts. Of particular interest with regard to heart disease is the ability of coconuts and coconut products to regulate insulin levels.

Insulin is a hormone that, among its other functions, helps your body make use of the energy it obtains from food. An increasing number of Americans today suffer from a condition known as insulin resistance due to such factors as poor diet, sedentary lifestyles, and being overweight. Insulin resistance is a metabolic disorder that occurs when the body's cells cannot properly take in enough insulin, thereby depriving the cells of energy. Insulin resistance has been linked to heart disease, especially among people who are also type 2 diabetics.

Your body's production of insulin is closely associated with blood sugar levels. High blood sugar negatively impacts insulin balance, leading to insulin resistance. The healthy fats found in coconut and its milk and oil play an essential role in regulating blood sugar. They do this by slowing down the body's digestive process of carbohydrate foods to ensure a steady, even supply of energy from such foods, which helps keep blood sugar levels steady. (Typically, blood sugar levels spike after carbohydrate foods are eaten because of how quickly the glucose they contain passes into the bloodstream.)

As you learned in Chapter 3, coconuts consist of medium-chain fatty acids (MCFAs), instead of the long-chain fatty acids found in vegetable oils. Unlike long-chain fatty acids, MCFAs are far better suited for energy use rather than fat storage. Whereas long-chain fatty acids can decrease cells' ability to absorb blood sugar, thereby causing or exacerbating insulin resistance, the MCFAs in coconuts have been shown to improve insulin sensitivity and glucose tolerance over time, and to increase the body's metabolic rate. An increased metabolism, in turn, helps to maintain proper functioning of insulin and to keep insulin levels balanced. Healthy metabolism is also very important when it comes to healthy heart function.

RESEARCH SHOWS SATURATED FATS ARE GOOD, FOR YOUR HEART, NOT BAD

As you learned in Chapter 3, the handful of studies that occurred decades ago that resulted in the American Heart Association and other health organizations, including agencies within the United States government, to warn against dietary saturated fat, as well as dietary cholesterol, were seriously flawed and the findings of those studies have subsequently been invalidated by more recent and better designed studies. Yet, as of this writing, the American Heart Association (AHA) continues to advise against consuming foods high in saturated fats, including coconuts and coconut oil. Millions of Americans today, as well as their doctors, continue to rely on the advice of the AHA. By doing so, they are failing to obtain the essential fatty acids that they need to stay healthy and prevent heart disease, as well as other serious conditions, including Alzheimer's and dementia (see Chapter 5).

Part of the problem is that many doctors and other health care experts today simply do not have time to keep abreast of the ongoing research that continues to establish the need for saturated fats in our diet, as well as the beneficial, heart-healthy effects such fats provide. Nor do most lay people. Nonetheless, the studies do exist and are readily available to be read by anyone who has the time and the desire to do so.

Let me draw your attention to a meta-analysis of saturated fats in relation to heart disease that was published in the *American Journal of Clinical Nutrition* in October, 2010. A meta-analysis is a scientific review of multiple studies that have previously been conducted on the same subject. According to the authors of the meta-analysis, its objective "was to summarize the evidence related to the association of dietary saturated fat with risk of coronary heart disease (CHD), stroke, and cardiovascular disease (CVD; CHD inclusive of stroke) in prospective epidemiologic studies."

Epidemiologic studies analyze the causes and effects of disease conditions in specific, well-defined populations, and also examine any patterns by the people within those populations that may be related to those causes and effects. The results of such studies are then usually used to shape public health decisions and policies because of how the studies identify risk factors for specific diseases.

For the meta-analysis mentioned above, researchers analyzed 21 previous studies. The studies in question ranged in length from 5 to 23 years of following up a total of 347,747 study participants to determine how many of them developed heart disease or stroke and what, if anything, their diets had to do with that development. During that time period, 11,006 study participants developed heart disease or stroke. However, according to the meta-analysis of these studies, dietary saturated fats "were not associated with an increased risk for CHD, stroke, or CVD." As a result of their meta-analysis, its authors concluded that "there is no significant evidence for concluding that dietary saturated fat is associated with an increased risk of CHD or CVD."

Following publication of this meta-analysis, Richard D. Feinman, professor of biochemistry and medical researcher at State University of New York Health Science Center at Brooklyn (also known as SUNY Downstate Medical Center), published an article in the medical journal *Lipids* entitled "Saturated Fats and Health: Recent Advances in Health." In that article he pointed out that, "Saturated fat of plant or animal origin has been an important ingredient in Western and non-Western diets for centuries," adding that "recommendations to reduce consumption persist *even in the face of equivocal or contradictory evidence* (emphasis added)."

He also wrote, "Although some long chain saturated fatty acids raise low-density (LDL) cholesterol in specific dietary interventions, these fatty acids may have a positive effect on the complex of other markers [such as] increased concentrations of small, dense LDL particles, decreased high-density lipoprotein (HDL) particles and increased triglycerides, which may be a more important risk factor for myocardial infarction and CVD.

"Finally," he concluded. "It is clear that regarding saturated fatty acids as one group is an over-simplification. Individual saturated fatty acids have specific functions depending on chain length. The relation between dietary intake of fats and health is complicated and the current publications point to the need to reduce over-simplification. Is it possible that evolution found benefits to saturated fatty acids that current recommendations do not consider?"

Given the mounting scientific evidence that continues to debunk claims that saturated fats, as well as dietary cholesterol by itself, are risk factors for heart disease, the answer to the question that Feinman posed at the end of his article appears to be a resounding Yes.

Despite this fact, the American Heart Association continues to advise the public to avoid saturated fats in favor of unsaturated fats, as evidenced by their 2017 Presidential Advisory *Dietary Fats and Cardiovascular Disease.* The AHA's stance on saturated versus unsaturated fats has remained the same since the AHA first warned against saturated fat intake and dietary cholesterol in 1961. In light of the scientific findings about saturated fats and dietary cholesterol, such as the ones above, I find the AHA's stance puzzling.

One of the studies that the AHA continues to cite as evidence that saturated fat increases the risk of heart disease (specifically atherosclerosis) was published in 1969 in the AHA's publication *Circulation.* In that study, which was limited only to men who were divided into two groups, one of which ate the standard high fat American diet of the time and the other of which ate a low fat diet that included vegetable oils, it was determined that the number of men who died of a heart attack was higher in those men who followed the standard high fat diet compared to the men in the low-fat diet group. What seems to be ignored by the AHA, however, is the fact that the total number of deaths by all causes was the same for both groups of men. Moreover, those who followed the low fat, vegetable oil diet died of cancer at twice the rate of the men in the high fat diet group. In addition, the researchers for this study concluded that the benefits that vegetable oil has for preventing atherosclerosis was due to the amount of vitamin E that vegetable oil used in the study contained, not the vegetable oil's polyunsaturated fat content.

Here are some other findings about saturated and unsaturated fats, as well as cholesterol, that have come to light in recent years:

- A scientific review published in the *British Medical Journal* in 2016 found that, while it is true that low saturated fat diet does indeed reduce cholesterol levels, researchers determined that lowering cholesterol in and of itself does not improve health outcomes, including the development of, or deaths caused by, cardiovascular disease. The authors of this scientific review concluded that "Available evidence from randomized controlled trials shows that replacement of saturated fat in the diet with linoleic acid [a type of unsaturated fat] effectively lowers serum cholesterol *but does not support the hypothesis that this translates to a lower risk of death from coronary heart disease or all causes* [italics added for emphasis]."

- A 2015 study published in the *American Journal of Clinical Nutrition* found that "Total fat intake was significantly associated with a lower risk of CVD [cardiovascular disease]" and that "Total fat intake was significantly associated with a lower risk of total death." The authors of this study also wrote, ""Most of the meta-analyses [of other studies] failed to show significant associations between the intake of SFAs [saturated fatty acids] and risk of CVD, stroke, or death."

  To be fair, the researchers of this study did find that pastries and other unhealthy foods high in saturated fats might increase the risk for heart disease, but that this is not the case for other high saturated fatty foods, such as fish, dairy products, and plant foods such as coconuts.

- Research dating back to at least the 1990s has found that saturated fats increases HDL "good" cholesterol levels. In addition, research has also shown that saturated fats also increase the size of so-called "bad" LDL cholesterol particles. This is very important, since smaller LDL particles, especially in combination with high levels of triglycerides, can increase the risk of heart disease by as much as 300 percent. Larger size LDL particles reduce this risk.

- Research from that same decade also demonstrated that low cholesterol levels caused by eating a low-fat diet resulted in a significant increased risk of depression in older men. This is hardly surprising, since, as you will learn in Chapter 5, the human brain and healthy brain functions depend on cholesterol and fat.

- In addition, medical studies have also shown that *men with low cholesterol levels (below 165 m/dL)* due to low fat diets are seven times more likely to die prematurely from unnatural causes, including suicide and accidents.

The authors of one such study wrote, "In several clinical trials of interventions designed to lower plasma cholesterol, reductions in coronary heart disease mortality have been offset by an unexplained rise in suicides and other violent deaths." Similarly, additional research has found that women with a total cholesterol below 195 mg/dL have a higher risk of death from all causes compared to women with higher cholesterol levels.

Even if the scientific evidence showed that saturated fats and dietary cholesterol did increase the risk of heart disease, which it does not, surely such findings would be outweighed by the overall premature mortality rates that low cholesterol causes.

- In 2014, the Mayo Clinic, one of the world's foremost medical research and treatment centers, published a position paper in its medical journal *Mayo Clinic Proceedings* which stated, "For many years we have been told that to prevent cardiovascular disease (CVD), we must lower our intake of saturated fatty acids (SFAs) and instead eat more carbohydrates and poly-unsaturated fatty acids (PUFAs). Backed up by the National Cholesterol Education Program, the National Institutes of Health, and the American Heart Association, the medical profession has promoted this idea eagerly, although the number of contradictory scientific reports is almost endless.

  There is in fact much evidence that doing the opposite is more relevant...There is no evidence *that a lower intake of SFA can prevent CVD and a high intake of PUFAs without specification may result in a high intake of omega-6, which is associated with many adverse health effects.* [italics added for emphasis] Because there is much evidence that saturated fat may even be beneficial, we urge the American Heart Association...to consider the aforementioned evidence when updating their future guidelines."

- In 2015, echoing the recommendation of the Mayo Clinic, the Dietary Guidelines Advisory Committee (DGAC) stated that dietary cholesterol should not be a concern because there is "no appreciable relationship between dietary cholesterol and serum cholesterol or clinical cardiovascular events in general populations." In their coverage of these new guidelines researchers writing in the *Journal of the American Medical Association* wrote, "The 2015 DGAC report tacitly acknowledges the lack of convincing evidence to recommend low-fat–high-carbohydrate diets for the general public in the prevention or treatment of any major health outcome, including heart disease, stroke, cancer, diabetes, or obesity."

These are only a small sampling of the many studies that call the saturated fat/high cholesterol myths regarding heart disease into question. Given such findings, it is my hope that the American Heart Association, as well as other organizations, including governmental health agencies, soon put a stop to the way they currently demonize both saturated fats and dietary cholesterol. By doing so, they could save countless lives.

Can Your Trust Your Heart Health to The American Heart Association?

The leading advocacy organization for the promotion of heart healthy advice is the American Heart Association (AHA). Formed in 1924 by six cardiologists, the AHA's mission is to "fight heart disease and stroke." Primarily a volunteer organization, the AHA today has over 30 million volunteers and supporters.

During its existence, there is no question that the AHA has done much to further our understanding of heart disease and stroke, helping many millions of people along the way. Many billions of dollars used to research heart disease and its prevention have been raised by the AHA throughout the years, and it is also the nation's largest provider of instruction in life-saving CPR techniques.

For all the heart-related pioneering research and medical techniques which the AHA has helped fund and for which we should all be grateful, there is one area of research in which the AHA seems to remain behind the times. Namely, the dietary advice it continues to recommend to prevent and to reverse heart disease. Most specifically, I am referring to the AHA's decades' long and indiscriminate advice against saturated fats and dietary cholesterol. As you read on page 61, even the prestigious Mayo Clinic is now calling this advice into question and urging the AHA to do away with it.

Why? Because the dietary guidelines the AHA recommends are outdated, erroneous, and potentially very harmful. Despite such urgings, as evidenced by its 2017 Presidential Advisory on Dietary Fats and Cardiovascular Disease, the AHA remains adamant that all saturated fats are unhealthy, while advocating for a low fat diet that includes unsaturated, not saturated oils and foods, and continuing to blame high cholesterol as a primary cause of heart disease. As I hope the information and studies I am sharing in this book make clear, the AHA's views on saturated and unsaturated fats, as well as on dietary cholesterol are not supported by recent scientific research.

Sadly, however, whenever the AHA issues reports or statements that demonize saturated fats and dietary cholesterol, its pronouncements are quickly taken up and spread by the mainstream media, not only in the United States, but around the world. And, in these days in which so many media companies, due to reduced staffing and lack of revenues, rely on "press release journalism," few journalists take the time to examine such pronouncements before parroting them to their respective audiences.

The AHA's 2017 Presidential Advisory is a case in point and a particularly curious one, at that. Because, once it was published, most media outlets in the U.S., as well as in Canada, the UK, and elsewhere, chose to focus their reporting on it in a way that damned coconut oil most of all. The headline that ran in *USA Today* on June 16, 2017 is a good example of what I mean. It proclaimed, "Coconut Oil Isn't Healthy, It's Never Been Healthy." Similar headlines that day and in the week that followed could be found in many other major newspapers and other media outlets.

What is most curious about these headlines is the fact that the AHA's advisory itself is 25 pages long (you can find it at the AHA's website, www.heart.org), yet contains only one paragraph of text specifically about coconut oil. Why, then, was coconut oil made the villain in media headline after headline? Could it be it's because the mainstream media today here in the United States relies so heavily on advertising dollars from both the pharmaceutical industry and major food companies? I cannot say.

Yet, what I can say is that both the pharmaceutical industry and many major food companies have a vested financial interest in maintaining the saturated fats/high cholesterol myth. In the case of Pharma, it is because of the many cholesterol-lowering statin drugs they promote, sales from which represent a significant portion of Pharma's annual revenues. And in the case of many major food companies, it is because their products are loaded with unsaturated fats from vegetable oils. At a time when even the AHA admits that 72 percent of all Americans regard coconut oil as a "healthy food," it is reasonable to assume that the consumer demand for coconut oil, and consumers' corresponding shift away from vegetable oils, as well as the ongoing research that continues to debunk the saturated fat/high cholesterol myth, all combine to threaten the profits of both Pharma and many major food groups.

But what do Pharma and major food groups have to do with the AHA's dietary recommendations?

Perhaps nothing, yet it just so happens that much of the funding for the AHA each year comes in the form of donations from some of the largest and most notable pharmaceutical and food companies in existence today. Corporate donors to the AHA include the Pharma companies AstraZeneca, Eli Lilly, Glaxo-Smith Kline, Merck, and Pfizer, among others. Major food companies that regularly donate to the AHA include General Mills, Kellogg's, Kraft, Nestle, and Pepsico. In addition, the AHA also receives donations from food lobby groups, such as Ag Canada and the Canola Oil Council, both of which have a vested interest in promoting unsaturated vegetable oils while demeaning saturated fats. In addition, the lead authors of the AHA's 2017 Presidential Advisory have all in the past received significant funding from various pharmaceutical companies and/or food lobbyist groups. Perhaps that is why these authors, as leading health journalist Gary Taubes and others pointed out following publication of the 2017 Presidential Advisory, cherry-picked the studies they chose to support their claims that saturated fats, including those from coconut oil, should be avoided. In fact, they primarily relied on only four studies, none of which was conducted after 1969.

Again, I cannot say why the authors of the Presidential Advisory wrote what they wrote, nor can I say why the AHA endorsed their claims.

Yet, as Upton Sinclair wrote many years ago, "It is difficult to get a man to understand something when his salary depends on his not understanding it." Unfortunately, the same holds true for organizations, such as the AHA that are dependent on outside funding. In any event, given its continued insistence that all saturated fats should be avoided or limited in one's diet, I recommend that you do not rely on American Heart Association when it comes to dietary advice. After all, not only does the AHA seem to have an obvious bias against saturated fats, including those from coconut oil, it is the same organization that for 30 years promoted margarine, which is loaded with trans fat and very similar to plastic in terms of its chemical composition, as a healthy alternative to butter.

COCONUTS HELP COMBAT THE MAJOR RISK FACTORS FOR HEART DISEASE

In addition to helping to support and maintain some of the most important components of a healthy heart, coconuts have been shown by research to play an equally important role in protecting against the most significant risk factors for heart disease, beginning with cholesterol and inflammation.

Oxidized Cholesterol

As Chapter 3 revealed, cholesterol, by itself, is not the threat to a healthy heart that most people, including physicians, continue to believe it to be. In large part, this belief in the high cholesterol model of heart disease persists because the American Heart Association and other health organizations continue to warn against high cholesterol. Yet, a growing body of research has established that cholesterol levels per se are not the problem. As you also learned in Chapter 3, without cholesterol your body simply could not function properly.

When cholesterol does become a threat, it does so because cholesterol, particularly LDL cholesterol, has become oxidized. As this oxidation process occurs it can result in persistent inflammation in the body, including within the arteries. Let's take a closer look as to why this is important.

Since the 1990s, a growing number of cardiologists and other physicians have begun moving away from the high cholesterol model of heart disease, recognizing its inherently flawed premise. In place of this model, they are shifting their focus onto chronic, low-grade inflammation, or the "inflamed artery" model.

Chronic Inflammation

There are two types of inflammation: acute and chronic. Acute inflammation occurs in response to trauma to the body, such as cuts, wounds, bruises, or acute (short-term) infection. Within seconds of such circumstances occurring, your body's immune response kicks in, creating a temporary inflammation response in order to speed immune cells, proteins, and other healing compounds to surround the affected area and begin the healing process. Once the acute trauma that causes this type of inflammatory response passes, so too does the response itself. Depending on the severity of the trauma, this type of acute immune response will stop within minutes, hours, or a few days. In contrast, chronic inflammation is characterized by an ongoing inflammatory response that, while less noticeable than that of an acute inflammatory response, can be damaging over time.

The theory that heart disease is caused by chronic inflammation is actually not new. In fact, it was first proposed in the 19th century by the physician regarded as the father of modern pathology, Dr. Rudolf Virchow. Dr. Virchow theorized that atherosclerosis, a common precursor to heart disease, was an inflammatory disease more than 150 years ago. But it was not until the late 20th century that physicians began to seriously consider chronic inflammation's role in heart disease. Two published scientific papers, in particular, played critical roles in this shift.

The first paper was a monograph published in 1998 by the American Heart Association and edited by its president, Valentin Fuster, M.D., Ph.D., Director of the Cardiovascular Institute at Mount Sinai School of Medicine, in New York City, which stated that 85 percent of all heart attacks and strokes were due to vulnerable plaque, a "soft" form of cholesterol, proteins, and blood cells that builds up within the arterial wall. The findings of the monograph were widely reported in both conventional medical journals and the mainstream media and debunked the belief that heart disease is primarily due to hard arterial plaque that obstructs the artery (the high cholesterol/blocked artery model). Given the fact that Dr. Fuster is the only cardiologist to receive four major research awards from the world's top four cardiovascular organizations (the AHA, the American College of Cardiology, the European Society of Cardiology, and the InterAmerican Society of Cardiology), the monograph proved quite influential.

As the monograph explained, vulnerable plaque primarily consists of soft cholesterol and clotting proteins that are different than the type of obstructing plaque common in atherosclerosis, and which is contained by a fibrous cap that is thinner and weaker than obstructing plaque and more easily ruptured. The body reacts to vulnerable plaque in much the same way that it deals with infection, releasing blood cells to attack and inflame the fibrous cap. This attack and the subsequent inflammation that results from it can cause the cap to break, spilling the powerful coagulants found in its interior into the bloodstream, where they can form large and lethal clots.

Cardiologists now believe that vulnerable plaque explains why some people with little or no blockages in their arteries can still have heart attacks, while others with almost completely blocked arteries may never experience any symptoms of heart disease. In the "inflamed artery" model of heart disease, plaque in the arteries is regarded as a mechanism the body uses to repair damage in the arterial walls. In response to such tears, the body releases various substances into the bloodstream to adhere, or stick, to the site of the tears. There, these substances attract a special class of cells called platelets, which are responsible for clotting, and together they combine to form the protective fibrous cap. It is the integrity of the cap itself that determines the stability of the plaque.

It is now recognized that oxidized cholesterol, as well as chronic infection, can trigger the formation of vulnerable plaque, setting in motion a vicious cycle, since the inflammation response is one of the ways your body deals with both oxidized cholesterol and infections. When vulnerable plaque comes in contact with oxidized cholesterol or infections, the body, in its attempt to prevent the further spread of these substances, causes the blood passing through the infected area to become hyper-coagulable and viscous. A clot may also form, impeding blood flow. Left untreated, this process can eventually result in heart disease and possibly death.

In 2002, another major scientific paper expanded the findings of the Fuster monograph, and truly laid the cornerstone for the emerging chronic inflammation/"inflamed artery" model of heart disease. Written by lead author Dr. Peter Libby, chief of cardiovascular medicine at the Brigham and Women's Hospital in Boston, MA and director of the D.W. Reynolds Cardiovascular Clinical Research Center at Harvard University, the paper appeared in the prestigious medical journal *Circulation*. Entitled *Inflammation and Atherosclerosis*, it proved to be a seminal article that has subsequently been cited in no less than 9,500 other scientific papers.

As Dr. Libby pointed out, atherosclerosis occurs when various white blood cells that act as the first line of defense against infectious agents take hold and become active in arterial tissue. At the onset of this process, small particles of LDL cholesterol begin to accumulate within the artery wall. As they do so, they start to be altered chemically. Then the modified LDL cholesterol triggers the artery's endothelial cells to release molecules that latch on to immune cells in the blood (primarily monocytes and T-cells). At the same time, the endothelial cells secrete chemicals called *chemokines* that entice the snared immune cells into the innermost layer of the artery's membrane structure.

Once inside this membrane structure, monocyte immune cells transform into macrophages that seek out and ingest the modified LDL cholesterol. As they do so, the macrophages fill up with fatty droplets until they are so laden with fat that they become what are known as foam cells. Meanwhile T cells also ensnared within the membrane start to form the earliest stages of plaque. Plaque buildup and growth is further promoted by other inflammatory molecules, triggering the formation of the fibrous cap that is characteristic of vulnerable plaque. This cap increases the size of the plaque while also walling it off from the blood. However, over time other inflammatory substances secreted by the foam cells weaken the cap and can cause it to rupture. Should such a rupture occur, dangerous blood clots can form, ultimately leading to a heart attack or a stroke.

Benefits of a Coconut-Rich Diet

So what does all of this have to do with coconuts and their milk and oil? Quite a lot. A coconut-rich diet can protect against heart disease in five very important ways.

1. First, unlike the fatty acids found in vegetable oils, the fatty acids in coconut food products are highly resistant to the oxidation process because of how stable they are. As a result, when they are consumed they do not create free radicals. By contrast, when unsaturated fats found in both mono- and polyunsaturated oils are consumed, they can quickly grow rancid inside the body, resulting in the proliferation of free radicals, which in turn trigger oxidation, including within the body's supply of cholesterol. (Remember, your body, in order to stay healthy, continuously produces its own supply of cholesterol in the liver.)

   It's long been established that a diet rich in antioxidant foods can prevent free radical damage and the oxidation process. Because of this, such a diet has also long been recommended for people who have or who are at risk of developing heart disease. The MCFAs found in coconut and its milk and oil, because of their high degree of stability and resistance to oxidation, act as antioxidants and have been shown to protect both cholesterol and unsaturated fats from becoming oxidized. As a result, regular consumption of coconut, coconut milk, and coconut oil can also help prevent the chronic inflammation that can lead to heart disease.

2. Another important benefit provided by coconuts with regard to heart disease is the positive effects it has on the so-called "bad" LDL cholesterol. As mentioned above, it is this form of cholesterol that builds up within the arterial walls as a result of the oxidation/inflammation process. By contrast, "good" HDL cholesterol has a beneficial effect on the arteries because of its ability to prevent the arteries from becoming blocked by plaque buildup.

   Research on coconut and the fatty acids it contains has consistently shown that its fatty acids, especially lauric acid, improves the HDL:LDL ratio by increasing HDL levels while simultaneously reducing LDL levels. In part, this is because coconuts' fatty acids can actually convert LDL cholesterol into HDL cholesterol. One reason for this is that coconuts' medium chain fatty acids are rapidly metabolized in the liver to produce energy instead of being used to manufacture and transport cholesterol.

   Just as importantly, coconut fatty acids also lowers levels of a particularly dangerous type of LDL cholesterol known as lipoprotein(a). This is significant because high levels of lipoprotein(a) can dramatically increase the risk of heart attack, stroke, and other types of heart disease. This has been confirmed by research, including a study of women that found that women who followed coconut-based diets, and who used non-hydrogenated coconut oil for food preparation, had lower levels of lipoprotein (a), based on blood tests taken after meals, compared to women who followed a low-saturated fat diet and who cooked with vegetable oils. Among all of the women in the coconut-based diet group, lipoprotein (a) was lowered because their diets were high in the saturated fats coconuts and coconut oil.

3. The third important reason why coconut, coconut milk, and coconut oil can help protect against heart disease is because coconuts' fatty acids have proven, powerful antimicrobial benefits and therefore help to reduce the level of infections in the body that lead to chronic inflammation. Ever since the inflammation model of heart disease was first discovered, a growing body of research has confirmed the role that chronic infection can play in the development and worsening of heart disease. This includes bacterial infections from the gums and mouth, which can migrate into the blood-stream to eventually negatively affect the heart and its arteries. You will learn more about the potent antimicrobial properties of coconuts, as well as its benefits for boosting your body's immune function in Chapter 6. While in Chapter 11 you will discover how the use of coconut oil can make a dramatic positive difference in the overall health of your mouth, gums, and teeth.

4. Because of the B vitamins they contain, adding coconuts to your diet can also provide a fourth important benefit for your heart and cardiovascular system. That's because B vitamins help to regulate and prevent elevated levels of homocysteine.

    Homocysteine is a naturally-occurring amino acid in the body, and is also obtained by eating protein-rich foods, especially meat. High levels of homocysteine in the body is today considered to be a risk factor for heart disease. The reason for this is because elevated homocysteine levels have been found to increase the likelihood of atherosclerosis (hardening of the arteries), as well as unhealthy blood clots, which can lead to stroke.

    The standard American diet, rightly known as SAD, is deficient in B vitamins, as well as many of the other nutrients coconuts contain (*see* Chapter 2). Making coconuts a part of your diet can help to rectify this problem, and also help keep your body's homocysteine levels under control. Not only that, but when you eat coconut with other foods during meals it slows down the time food takes to move out of the stomach during the digestion process. This, in turn, means that while in the stomach foods are exposed to the stomach's digestive enzymes for longer periods, helping to ensure that they are more completely metabolized so that the nutrients they contain can be better absorbed and more fully used by your body.

5. Finally, a coconut-rich diet also helps to keep blood pressure levels under control, preventing high blood pressure, which is another major risk factor for heart disease. The ways that coconuts help to safeguard against high blood pressure is discussed in Chapter 7.

One of the most significant studies that attests to the benefits coconuts, and especially coconut oil, have for heart health was conducted by researchers in Spain and published in 2015. The name of the study says it all: "A Coconut Extra Virgin Oil-Rich Diet Increases HDL Cholesterol and Decreases Waist Circumference and Body Mass in Coronary Artery Disease Patients."

The researchers of this study wrote that extra virgin coconut oil "has been acknowledged for its high proportion of medium-chain fatty acids (MCFAs), lauric acid (source of vitamin E), and polyphenols with antioxidant activity. The scientific literature has shown benefits of extra virgin coconut oil to the reduction of body fat, but there is still controversy over its effects on lipid [cholesterol] profile, since it is a source of saturated fat. Thus, the aim of this study was to evaluate the effect of a diet rich in coconut oil concerning the improvement of lipid profile and anthropometric [body fat composition] measurements."

The study involved 116 men and women, all of whom had a history of coronary artery disease (CAD), a type of heart disease that occurs in the arteries of the heart. In cases of CAD, the inner walls of the coronary arteries become diseased or damaged, causing plaque buildup within the arteries. This causes the coronary arteries to harden (atherosclerosis) and narrow, restricting blood flow and forcing the heart to work harder. Left untreated, CAD can cause sudden death as the heart simply stops working.

The participants in the study were between the ages of 45 and 85, with 70 percent of them being elderly. Approximately 63 percent of the participants were men. All of the participants suffered from high blood pressure and nearly all of them (94.5 percent) were on medication to control their cholesterol levels.

The study was conducted in two stages. During both stages, the authors of the study wrote, "Patients were seen in a monthly basis at the clinical nutrition department of a specialized hospital, where they received intensive dietary treatment with periodic phone calls to assess compliance. In addition, all patients were provided with a telephone number to contact to dispel doubts whenever necessary. Socioeconomic and demographic data, information on past medical history and present illness, drug therapy, and physical exercise were collected. In each visit, 12-hour fasting blood sample was drawn, 24-hour dietary recall was obtained, anthropometric [body fat composition] assessment was made and systemic blood pressure (BP) was measured."

The first stage of the study lasted for three months, during which time all of the participants received nutritional guidance and followed an "intensive" dietary nutritional treatment program. At the end of the first stage, all of the participants achieved a "significant decrease" in their overall weight, body mass index (BMI), neck circumference, waist circumference, and blood sugar profiles.

In the study's second stage, which lasted for another three to six months, depending on each person, the participants were divided into two groups. Both groups continued to follow the same dietary program of the first stage, but one of the groups was also given 13 mL (approximately one tablespoon) of extra virgin coconut oil to consume each day. The participants in this group were instructed to consume the coconut oil either alone or mixed with fruit, away from meals.

By the end of the study, the researchers found that the participants who consumed coconut oil each day during stage two were noticeably better able to maintain and further improve their weight loss, body mass index, and blood sugar profiles that both groups achieved in stage one, compared to the group that did not consume coconut oil. More importantly, the coconut oil group also exhibited increased levels of HDL ("good") cholesterol, as well as a statistically significant decrease in their waist circumference and, thus, belly fat, a major risk factor for heart disease. No such improvements were found in the non-coconut oil group.

"Dietary interventions that contribute to the increase of HDL concentrations are rare; therefore our findings were highly significant and unprecedented in this group of patients with chronic coronary disease," the authors of the study wrote.

Another important study that showcases the ability of coconuts to protect against heart disease is known as the Kitivan study. The study gets its name because it involved researching the health status of people in Kitiva, a South Pacific island that is part of Papua, New Guinea. In the traditional Kitivan diet, approximately 63 percent of all calories that the people consume are from saturated fats from coconuts. Coconut is a primary food staple in the traditional Kitivan diet, along with fruits, root vegetables (tubers) such as potatoes, and fish.

In the study, 213 adult natives of the island were interviewed to determine if they had experienced any warning signs of heart disease or stroke, such as chest pain, chest pain after physical exertion, and balance problems. They were also screened for aphasia (the inability to comprehend what others are saying and/or to speak intelligibly due to brain damage caused by stroke or other factors), and weakness on one side of the body (hemiparesis), another sign of stroke. None of the participants, who ranged in age from 20 to 96, reported any such symptoms. Most of the participants in this study (119 men and 52 women) were also given electrocardiograms (EKGs) to screen for undetected signs of a previous heart disease or stroke. No such signs were detected, despite the Kitivan's high saturated fat consumption. Based on this study, the researchers who conducted it wrote that the incidence of both stroke and heart disease "appear to be absent in this population."

The lead author of the Kitivan study was Staffan Lindeberg, MD, PhD, (1950 to 2016), an Associate Professor of Family Medicine at the Department of Medicine, University of Lund, Sweden. A year after he completed it, Dr, Lindeberg conducted a follow-up study in which he compared the cardiovascular risk factors among Kitivans who followed their traditional diet that is rich in coconuts and the saturated fats they contain with the same risk factors found in healthy populations in Sweden. In this study, Dr. Lindeberg and his colleagues tested 151 males and 69 females between the ages of 14 and 87. The cardiovascular health status of both the Swedish and Kitivan participants were analyzed by measuring their sitting systolic and diastolic blood pressure, their weight, height, and body mass index, the circumferences of their waist, pelvis and mid upper arm, their triceps skinfold thickness. They also analyzed their fasting serum total cholesterol, triglycerides, high-density lipoprotein cholesterol, estimated low-density lipoprotein cholesterol, apolipoprotein B, apolipoprotein A1 and apolipoprotein (a) levels, all of which are markers for heart disease.

What the study found was that, again, despite the high amount of calories that the Kitivan obtained each day in the form saturated fats from coconut, compared to the Swedes, their systolic and diastolic blood pressure, levels, body mass index, and triceps skinfold thickness "were substantially lower," as were their fasting serum total cholesterol, low-density lipoprotein cholesterol and apolipoprotein B levels. Based on these findings, Dr. Lindeberg and his colleagues wrote, "Of the analyzed variables, leanness and low diastolic blood pressure seem to offer the best explanations for the apparent absence of stroke and ischemic heart disease in Kitava. The lower serum cholesterol may provide some additional benefit. Differences in dietary habits may explain the findings." In other words, it is the Kitivans' traditional, coconut-rich diet that is the most likely reason that they do not suffer from heart disease or stroke.

Based on the results of the above studies and others like them, you can see why an increasing number of physicians and other health care providers no longer warn against the saturated fats that coconuts and coconut oil contain. Instead, they recommend the use of coconut oil to protect against heart disease and other health conditions because of the many benefits its MCFAs provide.

Addressing the Critics of the Kitivan Studies

A number of critics of the Kitivan studies often mistakenly conclude what the underlying reasons for the studies' results are. Some people assume the main reason the Kitivans are so healthy is that they eat a high fat, low carbohydrate diet. That isn't the case. As mentioned, the traditional Kitivan diet is certainly high in saturated fats because of its high coconut content. Yet it is also high in carbohydrates, including starchy carbohydrates from the root vegetables, and sugar from the fruits, the Kitivans regularly consume.

Given these facts, some critics assume that the Kitivans' exceptional health status is not due to their coconut consumption, but to their genes. Their assumption is that the people of Kitivan must be genetically predisposed to not be at risk for heart attack, stroke, and other types of heart disease. But once again the evidence proves that is not the case. Were genes the primary reason for the Kitivans' excellent cardiovascular health and overall health in general (they also have a very low incidence of other serious chronic diseases, including diabetes and Alzheimer's and dementia so long as they follow their traditional diet), their diet would not matter as much. Yet additional research has confirmed that their diet most definitely matters. Because when people from Kitiva, as well as people from other Pacific nations with similar traditional diets who also have a low incidence of heart disease and stroke, adopt a modern Western diet that is low in coconut and its saturated fats, within a generation they go on to develop heart disease, stroke, diabetes, and other chronic degenerative diseases at a comparable rate to what we experience here in the United States.

All of the above facts add further weight to the conclusions reached by researchers who have studied the Kitivans and other Pacific peoples. Namely, that the extremely low incidence of heart disease, stroke, and other conditions among their populations is primarily due to their coconut-rich traditional diets.

Other Tips for Keeping Your Heart Healthy

Adding coconuts, coconut milk, and coconut oil to your diet, of course, is hardly the only thing you need to do to keep your heart healthy. Although a full discussion on heart health is beyond the scope of this book, here are some other important tips that can help you protect your heart.

Diet

The food choices you make each day are one of the most important factors that determine how healthy you will be. For better heart and overall health, the best diet is one that is low in unhealthy fats (both trans fats as well as an excessive intake on omega-6 fatty acids that cause inflammation in the body). A diet low in sugar and simple carbohydrates, and rich in unprocessed, ideally organic, foods, including lean organ meats, fish, and plenty of fiber-rich fresh fruits and vegetables is ideal. Whole grains and legumes are also healthy, although research continues to find that even healthy carbohydrates should only be eaten in moderation. Also be sure to drink plenty of pure filtered water throughout the day, as well as fresh coconut milk or water if it is available. And for cooking and baking purposes, use extra virgin coconut oil.

Exercise

Regular exercise is also important. However, contrary to popular opinion, exercise does not have to be intense or prolonged in order for you to benefit from it. In fact, prolonged periods of intense exercise has now been found to increase inflammation levels in the body. For best results, choose a type of exercise or physical activity you enjoy, such as a regular daily 20 minute walk, bicycling, or swimming.

Lifestyle

Adopting a healthy lifestyle is also vitally important. This means not smoking and avoiding secondhand smoke and limiting your intake of caffeine and alcohol drinks (especially hard alcohol; one or two glasses of beer or red wine each day is not only permissible but also good for your heart). Losing weight, if you need to do so, is also important (you will learn how coconuts can help you do so in Chapter 8).

Overall, a healthy lifestyle is one in which you avoid the lifestyle choices above and replace them with heart healthy meals and regular physical activity, along with engaging in other activities you enjoy, such as a favorite hobby, which can promote relaxation and increase enjoyment. Also make it a point to spend quality time with your family and friends. Such healthy lifestyles choices will also help you to better cope with stress, which is also vitally important given how closely associated chronic stress is with heart disease.

CONCLUSION

As this chapter makes clear, despite all of the marvelous advances that have been made to detect and treat it, heart disease continues to be our nation's number one killer. However, by understanding the major risk factors discussed in this chapter that cause heart disease, it is my hope that you now understand there is much you can do on your own to protect yourself and your loved ones from experiencing heart attack, stroke, and other types of heart disease. I hope you also now understand how and why adding coconuts to your diet, including cooking and baking with coconut oil instead of other oils, can be a wise and delicious choice for maintaining a healthy heart.

Now let's explore the ways in which coconuts can help protect and enhance the functioning of your body's other most important organ—your brain. That is the focus of Chapter 5.

5.

Coconuts and Your Brain

Your brain is what makes you human. It has shaped your personality, provided you with the capacity to read and understand these words and master your language. It has given you the capacity to think, decide, distinguish right from wrong, create, and interact and successfully cope with the outside world. Your brain also controls every function in your body, from your ability to breathe and move, to orchestrating and overseeing all of the untold, moment-to-moment processes carried out by your body's trillions of cells. Without your brain, you could not process and make sense of the constant stream of sensory data that bombards your senses each and every moment of your life, including when you are sleeping, nor could you remember and learn from your past experiences and memories, every single one of them having been recorded by your brain's neurons.

Yet, like your heart, today your brain is under more assaults than ever before, which is why in recent decades there has been a frightening surge in the incidence of brain diseases, such as Alzheimer's and dementia. As with many other degenerative diseases, such types of brain disease were once rare. Now, they are not only becoming commonplace, they are manifesting earlier than ever before. Where only a few short decades ago conditions such as Alzheimer's and dementia seemed to manifest only in old age, today they are afflicting otherwise seemingly healthy men and women in their 50s and, in some cases, even earlier. Consider these facts:

- One in eight Americans 65 and older has Alzheimer's disease.

- Forty-five percent of all Americans 85 and older have Alzheimer's.

- Nearly five percent of all Americans below the age of 65 are also afflicted with Alzheimer's.

- Alzheimer's disease is the sixth leading cause of death in the United States.

The statistics on dementia among Americans is equally grim, with the incidence of dementia projected to double every 20 years. (*Dementia* is an umbrella term used to describe a variety of diseases and conditions that develop when nerve cells in the brain die or no longer function normally. The death or malfunction of these nerve cells, called neurons, causes changes in one's memory, behavior, and ability to think clearly. These changes eventually impair the brain's ability to properly oversee such basic bodily functions as walking and swallowing.)

It is commonly assumed that the rise in Alzheimer's and dementia rates are primarily due to the fact that, overall, Americans are living longer than their ancestors. That assumption is erroneous. There are far more important

Fascinating Facts About Your Brain

The adult human brain weighs approximately three pounds (1.4 kilograms), which is no more than two percent of the total body weight for most adult men. In appearance it resembles a mass of jelly.

On average, brains in adult males are approximately 10 percent larger than female brains even after the larger body size of males compared to females is taken into account. The larger brain size in men is not an indication of superior brain function, however. If brain size correlated to superior brain function, then our Neanderthal ancestors would have been better equipped than we are to face the modern world, since their brains were 10 percent larger than ours are. In fact , our brains are continuing to become smaller, with scientists estimating that human brain size has shrunk by the size of a tennis ball over the past 10 to 20,000 years.

In order to function properly your brain requires lots of oxygen and energy. It uses 20 percent of your body's total daily energy and oxygen supply.

Although most people think their brains are solid, in reality, like the rest of the human body, the brain is mostly composed of water, which comprises approximately 73 percent of the brain's mass. For this reason, chronic low-grade dehydration can impair healthy brain function, affecting memory and other cognitive skills.

The rest of your brain is comprised mostly of fats and proteins, with 60 percent of its solid mass made up of fats, making your brain the fattiest organ in your body. Healthy brain function depends on a regular supply of healthy fats, including saturated fats, in your diet.

One quarter (25 percent) of the cholesterol produced by your body ends factors involved that can take hold many years, and even decades, prior to symptoms of such conditions first becoming noticeable. Recognizing and addressing those factors before they become severe is the key to keeping your brain healthy and youthful.

Fortunately, your brain is one of the most adaptable and resilient organs in your body. When provided with what it needs to be healthy, it can exhibit remarkable powers of regeneration and renewal. In this chapter, you will discover some of the major factors that pose a threat to the health of your brain, and learn why dietary coconut, especially in the form of coconut oil, can help to prevent and alleviate the problems these risk factors pose.

---

up in the brain because cholesterol is an essential component of every brain cell. Without enough cholesterol brain cells will die. High total cholesterol levels have also been shown to reduce the risk of dementia and Alzheimer's disease.

There are an estimated 86 billion brain cells in the human brain, but not all brain cells are alike, and there are approximately 10,000 different types of neurons in the brain. Each neuron connects with an average of 40,000 synapses, with all neurons and synapses communicating with each other.

The human brain does not fully mature until around 25 years of age. Until recently, it was thought that once full brain maturity was achieved, the brain's neural pathways were set for the rest of one's life and no new neural pathways were capable of being formed. Scientists now know this is not true. New neural pathways can be formed at any age so long as the brain remains healthy. The brain's ongoing ability to form new neural pathways is known as *neuroplasticity.*

Your brain generates electricity, producing an average of 12 to 25 watts of electricity per day, which is enough energy to power a low-watt LED light bulb.

Over 100,000 chemical reactions occur within your brain every second.

Within your brain there are approximately 400 miles of blood vessels.

Contrary to popular opinion, we do not use only 10 percent of our brains. Brain scans reveal that we use almost all parts of our brains all of the time, including when we are sleeping.

Although your experience of pain is processed by the brain, the brain itself is incapable of feeling pain because it has no pain receptors, unlike all other organs in your body.

RISK FACTORS THAT
CAN DAMAGE YOUR BRAIN

The human brain, like the human body itself, is designed to be resilient in the face of the various challenges that present themselves during our existence on this planet. But when faced with persistent risk factors your brain can become overburdened and eventually, if these risk factors are not properly dealt with and reversed, impaired brain function will result. What follows is an overview of some of the most common factors that can negatively affect brain health.

Poor Diet and Nutritional Deficiencies

Poor diet and nutritional deficiencies are a primary cause of brain degeneration. Deficiencies in various vitamins, minerals, essential fatty acids, and amino acids, including those found in coconuts, coconut milk and water, and coconut oil, have all been linked to impaired brain function, as well as brain diseases, including Alzheimer's and dementia. These deficiencies are compounded by unhealthy diets, which not only prevent your brain from getting all of the nutrients it needs, but also result in over-acidity, chronic inflammation, and blood sugar imbalances.

One of the main reasons why a healthy diet and a daily supply of nutrients are so essential for proper brain function has to do with how the brain operates. It does so primarily through the transmission of chemical messengers known as neurotransmitters, which are responsible for how the brain communicates with the rest of the body. For neurotransmitters to be able to transmit the brain's messages effectively, an adequate supply of brain nutrients is necessary. When the supply of nutrients is insufficient, the brain and its functions are adversely affected.

ENVIRONMENTAL TOXINS

It is well known that environmental toxins play a significant role in various neurological conditions, in addition to other degenerative diseases, such as cancer, diabetes, and heart disease. Environmental toxins harm the brain both directly, by crossing the blood-brain barrier, and indirectly, by compromising immune and liver function. Toxins that cross the blood-brain barrier deposit themselves within brain tissues, causing brain cells, tissues, and neurotransmitters to become impaired. Eventually it leads to the buildup of brain plaque, which is a major contributing factor in the onset of Alzheimer's and dementia. This process is further exacerbated by the negative effects toxins have on the immune system and the liver.

Altered immune function caused by environmental toxins causes the blood-brain barrier to become more porous, or "leaky," in much the same way that toxins can cause leaky gut syndrome. The more porous the blood-brain barrier becomes, the easier it is for toxins to cross it and settle in brain tissue.

Blood Sugar Imbalances

Stable blood sugar (glucose) levels are essential for healthy brain function. Blood sugar levels that are too high (hyperglycemia), too low (hypoglycemia), or which regularly fluctuate between levels that are high and low, can all impair your brain's ability to perform its many tasks.

The reason blood sugar levels are such vital factors in brain health is because glucose is the brain's primary source of fuel. Optimal blood sugar levels help ensure that overall brain chemistry remains balanced, and also prevent damage to, or loss of, neuron structure and function, as well as the death of neurons. Balanced blood sugar levels are also required for the proper production of neurotransmitters, as well as healthy neurotransmitter metabolism and function.

Imbalanced, or unstable, blood sugar levels either deprive the brain of enough glucose or flood it with too much glucose. Either way, brain health is negatively impacted. Brain symptoms caused or made worse by low blood sugar include excess production of the adrenal hormones epinephrine and norepinephrine, as a result of low levels of the adrenal hormone cortisol. Cortisol, as mentioned earlier, prevents low blood sugar. Other symptoms caused by low blood sugar include mood swings, anxiety, irritability, forgetfulness, and feelings of lightheadedness.

High blood sugar levels result in insulin resistance, as the pancreas continues to produce insulin in an effort to force glucose into the cells. However, the excess glucose gets converted into fat, increasing total body fat. The conversion of glucose into fat requires energy, which creates adrenal fatigue. High insulin levels cause chronic inflammation, disruption of other hormones, and impaired neurotransmitter function, all of which, in turn, can cause degeneration of the brain and its functions. In addition, elevated blood sugar and insulin resistance also causes excessive production of cortisol.

Brain Inflammation

Another significant cause of impaired brain function is brain inflammation, also known as neuroinflammation. Just as chronic inflammation in the rest of your body can cause a wide range of health problems, it can also trigger brain and cognitive problems. As a matter of fact, inflammation in the brain and elsewhere in the body creates a vicious circle. A growing body of research is confirming a correlation between impaired brain health, chronic inflammation, and autoimmune responses in which the body's immune system attacks healthy tissues and organs. Studies have also linked brain inflammation to chronic depression.

When inflammation in the brain occurs, the rate at which neurons fire slows down. This, in turn, can lead to brain fog and impaired memory. Brain inflammation also reduces energy production in brain cells. Chronic brain inflammation can lead to neuron death and the onset of neurodegenerative diseases.

Oxygen Supply

A sufficient supply of oxygen to the brain is one of the most important requirements for healthy brain function. As it happens, oxygen deprivation lasting more than five minutes is all that is usually necessary to cause permanent brain damage. Signs of a lack of brain oxygen include poor focus and concentration, cold extremities (hands and feet), poor finger- and toenail health, and fungal growth on the toes.

Most of us typically believe we are getting all of the oxygen we need simply because we are still breathing. However, most people are habitually shallow breathers and are thus deprived of an adequate supply of oxygen on a daily basis.

Oxygen is carried to your brain by your blood, which also transports the nutrients, hormones, and neurotransmitters that your brain requires. Poor blood flow, or circulation, is the primary cause of lack of oxygen in the brain, and also the cause of vascular dementia, which is the second most common form of dementia after Alzheimer's disease. Lack of oxygen also prevents brain neurons from producing all of the energy they need to survive and carry out their many functions. In short, poor circulation and lack of oxygen to the brain go hand and hand.

Hormone Imbalances

Healthy hormone function is also essential for a healthy, optimally-functioning brain. Both brain neurons and various brain cells have receptor sites for hormones. Research has shown that healthy hormone balance plays important roles in preventing brain inflammation and degeneration, as well as in helping neural networks to grow and branch out, and in maintaining optimal neuroplasticity. Hormones also help to maintain the shape and structure of the brain. Hormone imbalances can seriously impair all of the above functions, as well as accelerate premature aging of the brain.

Pharmaceutical Drugs

The ongoing use of pharmaceutical drugs is one of the primary causes of dementia and other brain conditions, including delirium, in the elderly. This is especially true of people who have been prescribed more than one drug at a time. This is known as drug-induced cognitive impairment.

Given how widespread the use of pharmaceutical drugs has become in our society, drug-induced brain problems no longer affect just the elderly. This is not surprising, since all pharmaceutical drugs carry some risk of side effects. Common side effects related to the brain that can be caused by regular drug use also include anxiety, "brain fog," depression, erratic behavior patterns, and suicidal thoughts. In certain cases, drugs, either alone or used in combination, can even cause brain damage.

Many drugs can also interfere with the brain's ability to produce energy because of how they impair mitochondria function. Mitochondria act as your cells' energy plants. Among the highest concentrations of mitochondria in the body are those within the brain and the heart.

Another area of concern regarding brain health is the potentially harmful role that statin drugs may play. Statins, which act to lower cholesterol levels in the body, represent the most widely prescribed class of drugs in the U.S. today. As you learned in chapters 3 and 4, cholesterol of itself is not a risk factor for heart disease. Cholesterol plays many important roles in helping the body to maintain its health, including within the brain and the nervous system.

One of the most important roles cholesterol plays is in the formation of synapses, or connections between neurons. Synapse formation is directly dependent on cholesterol, and without enough cholesterol proper learning and memory function cannot take place. Actually, one of the reasons that healthy sleep is beneficial to learning and memory is because it enables the brain to make more cholesterol. Because of how statins inhibit cholesterol levels, a number of health experts speculate that the rising rates of Alzheimer's and dementia over the past few decades may, at least indirectly, be related to the corresponding increase in statin use over that same time period.

If you are currently using prescription drugs and suspect they may be affecting your brain function, speak with your doctor. In almost all cases normal brain function can be reversed or returned to its pre-drug state by stopping the use of the offending drug. The weaning off process needs to be supervised by a physician.

Lack of Sleep

As it is for the rest of your body, sleep is the time of repair for your brain. During sleep, your brain also consolidates the memories of what you learned and experienced during the day. Sleep also aids your brain in ridding itself of wastes.

Numerous previous studies have demonstrated how important healthy sleep is for brain health, and how lack of, or fitful, sleep can negatively impact the brain and its many functions. Lack of sleep has also been found to be a contributing factor in the development of Alzheimer's and dementia. Therefore, ensuring that you obtain adequate amounts of quality sleep each night is vitally important for maintaining optimal brain health.

COCONUTS TO THE RESCUE

Adding coconuts to your diet can help minimize many of the above risk factors that are known to harm the brain and impair brain functioning.

Nutritional Support

The first way in which coconuts can help has to do with the rich variety of nutrients coconuts contain, many of which are known to help maintain and improve brain health and brain function. As you learned in Chapter 2, coconuts supply a wide range of amino acids, many of which are known to enhance brain health, support the central nervous system, and help maintain the health of the brain's neurotransmitters. Of particular importance in this regard are the amino acids aspartic acid, cystine, glutamic acid, glycine, histadine, phenylalanine, serine, threonine, and tyrosine, all of which are found in coconuts. In addition, coconuts also supply the amino acids isoleucine and leucine, both of which help regulate blood sugar levels, as well as tryptophan, which helps support healthy sleep.

Coconuts also contain B vitamins, vitamin C, and the minerals magnesium, selenium, and zinc, which also play vital roles in supporting proper brain functioning and overall brain health. But perhaps the biggest nutritional benefits coconuts provide the brain are its rich supply of essential fats that are especially important for brain health. As mentioned above, healthy brain function depends on a regular supply of such healthy fats.

One of the benefits of the medium-chain fatty acids (MCFAs) found in coconut is that they bypass the body's digestive process, meaning that they are quickly absorbed by the body and made available for use, including in the brain. Once they enter the brain the MCFAs go to work helping to improve brain focus, counteract mental fatigue, and, along with the amino acids coconuts contain, act as fuel for the brain's neurotransmitters. Coconut MCFAs can also improve your mood and ward off feelings of anxiety and depression because of their ability to boost serotonin levels in the brain. In addition, the type of fats found in coconuts are a rich source of ketones, which are discussed in more detail on page 86.

Protection Against Brain Toxins

The nutrients contained in coconuts can protect the brain from toxins in two ways. First, as they do with all other cells in the body, the MCFAs in coconuts help to maintain the shape and integrity of brain cell membranes. This, in turn, helps to prevent toxins from passing through the membranes into the brain cells themselves.

The nutrients found in coconuts also play important roles in helping the body, including the brain, to detoxify, as well as protecting against a wide array of toxins and the free radical damage toxins can cause. In addition, the MCFAs in coconuts stimulate the activation of a special class of proteins known as *brain-derived neurotrophic factors* (BDNFs). These BDNF proteins aid in the production and repair of brain cells and help to eliminate toxins in the brain.

Blood Sugar Regulation

Blood sugar imbalances occur as a result of insulin spikes following meals, and the consumption of foods with a high glycemic index. The glycemic index is used to measure foods' effects on blood glucose (sugar) levels. Foods with a high glycemic index score increase blood sugar levels and insulin spikes. Adding coconuts and especially coconut oil to your meals can help regulate blood sugar levels and prevent insulin spikes.

Not only do coconuts and coconut oil have a very low glycemic index, they can also help to minimize the effects of high glycemic index foods because of how they slow the passage of such foods from the stomach. By doing so, coconuts and coconut oil reduce the rate in which glucose from such foods enter the bloodstream, preventing blood sugar spikes. Both coconuts and coconut oil also have a positive effect on insulin secretion by the body and help reduce problems associated with insulin sensitivity. These benefits are especially important for people who are overweight (*see* Chapter 8) and/ or who suffer from diabetes.

Protection Against Inflammation

As you learned in Chapter 4, the MCFAs found in coconut and its milk and oil, as well as some of the other nutrients they contain, act as antioxidants. They protect against free radical damage that can trigger and exacerbate levels of inflammation in the body, including in the brain. As a result, regular consumption of coconut, coconut milk, and coconut oil can also help prevent the chronic inflammation that can impair brain function and damage brain cells. The BDNF proteins activated by coconut's MCFAs also help to prevent and reduce brain inflammation.

In addition, the nutrients coconuts contain have powerful immune-enhancing properties. They can protect against harmful bacteria, fungi, viruses, and other microorganisms, all of which can cause inflammation in the body and the brain. You will learn more about the immune-boosting properties of coconuts in Chapter 6.

Hormone Balance

The combination of fatty acids and amino acids that coconuts contain has also been found to benefit the body's endocrine system by helping to regulate and stabilize hormone production. Among the hormones positively affected by coconuts are estrogen, serotonin, testosterone, and thyroid hormones. In large part coconut's benefits for hormone balance stems from how coconut increases beneficial HDL cholesterol levels, as well as its ability to convert so-called "bad" LDL cholesterol into HDL cholesterol. Healthy cholesterol is essential for the adequate production of your body's hormones.

Better Sleep

Although coconuts are not a sleep aid per se, indirectly they can help improve sleep because of the ability of the nutrients they contain to regulate blood sugar and insulin (blood sugar and insulin spikes can impair your ability to get a good night's sleep) and produce sleep hormones such as serotonin. As the quality of your sleep improves, so too will your brain function.

BENEFITS OF KETONES IN COCONUTS

A growing body of scientific research indicates that one of the primary reasons coconuts and coconut oil can help maintain the health of the brain has to do with the ketones they contain. Ketones are chemical substances that are produced when your body breaks down fat in order to produce energy. They are ordinarily produced when blood glucose levels become low. Glucose is the primary source of energy in both your body and your brain. In the event that your blood glucose levels fall, your body will draw upon its fat stores to produce ketones to supply and maintain its energy levels.

One of the primary uses of ketones in the body is to "feed" the brain by keeping it supplied with energy. In addition, ketones are able to pass through the blood brain barrier. Once inside the brain, they act as a neuroprotectant. They have also been shown to stimulate the growth of new brain cells to replace dead or dying cells. Besides being produced from fats in the body, ketones are also found in medium chain fatty acids (MCFAs). Coconuts, coconut oil, and coconut milk are especially rich sources of these MCFAs.

Typically, your body does not rely on ketones to produce energy because its primary energy source is the glucose that comes from the foods you eat. Your brain, as well, primarily relies on glucose for its own production of energy. However, too much glucose in the body can result in a variety of serious health problems, ranging from high blood sugar issues, diabetes and obesity, to an increased risk of both cancer and heart disease due to the insulin spikes that occur following consumption of high-glucose foods.

NEW HOPE FOR ALZHEIMER'S/DEMENTIA PATIENTS

Researchers have now also linked excess consumption of glucose-rich foods (starchy carbohydrates, sweets, and certain fruits that are high in sugar, such as bananas) with brain conditions, as well, ranging from temporary experiences of "brain fog" to chronic conditions, such as dementia and Alzheimer's disease. In fact, because of close association between a habitual consumption of foods high in glucose with the development of Alzheimer's disease, a growing number of neurologists and other physicians today refer to Alzheimer's as "type 3 diabetes." This is due to the fact that the same type of mechanisms that cause type 2, or adult-onset, diabetes also play a major role in the cognitive decline characterized by Alzheimer's and dementia. For this reason, more and more doctors today are urging their patients to limit their daily consumption of starchy carbohydrate foods and sugar-rich fruits, and to avoid sweets, sodas, and other sugary drinks altogether in order to reduce their risk of developing Alzheimer's and dementia, as well as cancer, diabetes, and heart disease.

Ironically, despite the brain's need for glucose to produce energy, regularly consuming foods with high glucose content can eventually result in a state in which the brain can no longer make use of glucose for its energy supply. This is precisely what happens in cases of Alzheimer's disease and dementia. In such conditions the brain itself begins to block its uptake of glucose. As this occurs, it creates a vicious circle in which the brain becomes deprived of energy, which in turn results in an overall state of brain degeneration, leading to further progression of these diseases.

Supplying the brain with ketones from coconuts and coconut oil can help prevent this problem from occurring, and may even help to reverse it. This provides new hope for people who are already suffering with Alzheimer's and dementia and for those who are at risk of developing such conditions. A dietary approach known as the "ketogenic diet," which consists of healthy, high fat foods, such as those found in coconuts and its oil, moderate protein

Ketoacidosis

Ketosis is sometimes confused with *ketoacidosis,* a potentially life-threatening condition that most often develops in people suffering with type 1 diabetes if they are unable to receive an insulin injection. As its name implies, ketoacidosis is a condition characterized by too much acidity in the body, specifically in the bloodstream. It is caused when blood sugar and ketone levels in the blood become too high due to a lack of insulin. Left untreated, ketoacidosis can damage liver and kidney function, and if it is not treated promptly, it can lead to coma and even death.

Normally, keotacidosis is prevented from occurring because of the body's ability to produce insulin, but people with type 1 diabetes are unable to produce sufficient amounts of insulin. Even most people with type 2 diabetes that is so severe that they need to inject insulin usually produce enough insulin of their own to prevent ketoacidosis from occurring.

intake, and low carbohydrate foods also offers promise in this area. Such a diet shifts the body into a state known as *ketosis.* In this state the body starts to produce energy from its stores of fats (specifically the ketones that the fats contain) rather than from the normal process of glycolysis, in which the body produces energy from glucose.

One of the leading researchers in the area of ketosis as an aid to Alzheimer's and dementia is Samuel T. Henderson, MD, Vice President of Research and Development at Accera, Inc., a biotechnology company focused on the development of therapies for brain and central nervous system disorders, including Alzheimer's and dementia. Dr. Henderson has authored and co-authored a number of published scientific studies that document the benefits that ketosis and a ketogenic diet can have for such conditions. In one of his published studies, Dr. Henderson pointed out that there are two mechanisms that are involved in the primary cause of Alzheimer's disease. Of these mechanisms, he wrote, "(1) Disturbances in lipid [fat] metabolism within the central nervous system inhibits the function of membrane proteins such as glucose transporters and the amyloid precursor protein. (2) Prolonged excessive insulin/IGF signaling accelerates cellular damage in cerebral neurons. These two factors ultimately lead to the clinical and pathological course of AD [Alzheimer's disease]. This hypothesis also suggests several preventative and treatment strategies. A change in diet emphasizing decreasing dietary carbohydrates and increasing essential fatty acids (EFA) may effectively prevent AD. Interventions that restore lipid [fat] homeostasis may treat the disease, including drugs that increase fatty acid metabolism, EFA repletion therapy, and ketone body treatment."

In another study authored by Dr. Henderson, he wrote, "An early feature of Alzheimer's disease (AD) is region-specific declines in brain glucose metabolism. Unlike other tissues in the body, the brain does not efficiently metabolize fats; hence the adult human brain relies almost exclusively on glucose as an energy substrate [source of energy]. Therefore, inhibition of glucose metabolism can have profound effects on brain function. The hypometabolism [low metabolism] seen in AD has recently attracted attention as a possible target for intervention in the disease process. One promising approach is to supplement the normal glucose supply of the brain with ketone bodies (KB) . . . KB are normally produced from fat stores when glucose supplies are limited, such as during prolonged fasting. KB have been induced both by direct infusion and by the administration of a high-fat, low-carbohydrate, low-protein, ketogenic diets. Both approaches have demonstrated efficacy in animal models of neurodegenerative disorders and in human clinical trials, including AD trials. Much of the benefit of KB can be attributed to their ability to increase mitochondrial efficiency [the ability of the mitochondria, the cells' "energy factories," to efficiently produce adequate amounts of energy] and supplement the brain's normal reliance on glucose. Research into the therapeutic potential of KB and ketosis represents a promising new area of AD research."

Other studies have confirmed that supplying people with ketones from fatty acids, such as those from coconut oil, can offer significant benefits for people suffering from Alzheimer's disease. One of the more noteworthy of these studies, which was co-authored by Dr. Henderson, was published in the medical journal *Neurobiology of Aging* in 2004. The study involved 20 patients suffering from either Alzheimer's disease or mild cognitive impairment. On alternating days the patients were given either ketone-rich MFCAs mixed with heavy whipping cream or heavy whipping cream alone as a placebo. The dose of MFCAs was 40 ml, which is the equivalent of slightly more than two and a half tablespoons of MFCA. The study found that a single dose of MFCAs improved the cognitive function of all 20 patients as determined by their improved ability to recall the information from texts they were asked to read. In addition, four of the test patients also exhibited improved performance on the Alzheimer's Disease Assessment Scale-Cognitive Subscale (ADAS-cog). According to Dr. Henderson and his co-authors of this study, these cognitive improvements were due to a corresponding increase in the patients' blood ketone levels. Blood testing was done before the patients were

given the MCFA mixture or the placebo, and then 90 minutes after the mixture of MCFAs or placebo were administered. The patients then underwent
a 30-minute cognitive testing session, after which their blood ketone levels
were again measured.

How Ketones in MCFAs Help to Enhance Brain Function

As mentioned, normally your brain is supplied with energy from the glucose
obtained from food. However, in order for the brain to make use of glucose for
its energy needs it must first process glucose using insulin. Recent research,
in fact, has found that the brain actually produces its own supply of insulin
in order to process glucose for energy. But as we age, the ability of the brain
to process glucose to meet its energy needs, as well as to repair damaged
brain cells, can diminish over time. This is one of the factors involved in the
onset and progression of Alzheimer's, dementia, and other cognitive-decline
conditions. Ketones supplied by MCFAs, such as those found in coconuts
and coconut oil, provide the brain with energy without the need for insulin
because of how readily accessible they are as an energy source.

The reason ketones in MCFAs go to work so quickly to produce energy in
the brain, as well as in the body in general, is because, unlike glucose, as well
as long chain fatty acids, MCFAs are rapidly metabolized in the liver when
they are consumed instead of being stored in the body as fat. This makes them
a readily accessible source for ketone production in the body. When insulin
resistance and impaired metabolism develop in the brain, its structure and
functioning can also become impaired. Ketones bypass the need for insulin to
quickly begin helping to improve the brain's metabolic processes and cognitive function. Ketones also stimulate blood flow to the brain which enhances
circulation and the delivery of oxygen to brain cells, further improving overall brain function.

And it's not only Alzheimer's and dementia for which ketones from
MCFAs offer promise in the brain. MCFAs, particularly caprylic acid, act as
natural anticonvulsants, and researchers have shown that caprylic acid can
help control convulsions caused by epileptic seizures. Animal studies using
caprylic acid indicate that it may also offer hope for people suffering from
Lou Gehrig's disease (ALS). In one such study conducted on mice the results
were so impressive that the researchers stated that caprylic acid could potentially be used to have "a high impact on the quality of life of ALS patients."

Because coconut oil is a rich source of caprylic acid, as well as other
ketone-producing MCFAs, research into the use of coconut oil to treat and prevent brain conditions has begun to grow in recent years. One such study was
conducted by researchers from the Memorial University of Newfoundland,

in Canada. They conducted a pilot study to investigate the effects of coconut oil supplementation directly on cortical neurons treated with amyloid-[beta] (A[beta]) peptide in vitro (outside of the body in an artificial environment). A[beta] peptide is the primary element in certain deposits found in the brains of patients with Alzheimer's disease and is believed to contribute to its onset and progression.

In the study, the researchers exposed live rat neurons to various combinations of A[beta] peptide and coconut oil. The A[beta] peptide alone reduced the survival time of the neurons, while the coconut oil protected the neurons against the A[beta] peptide and increased the neurons' survival time. The researchers observed that A[beta]-cultured neurons treated with coconut oil appeared "healthier," and that the coconut oil "rescued" the neurons from damage within the neuron's mitochondria caused by the A[beta] peptide's toxicity. Coconut oil was also found to prevent changes in the size and shape of the mitochondria that would otherwise have been caused by the A[beta] peptide. These findings are important because mitochondria function is typically impaired in the brains of Alzheimer's disease patients.

Based on their findings, the researchers stated, "The rationale for using coconut oil as a potential AD therapy is related to the possibility that it could be metabolized to ketone bodies that would provide an alternative energy source for neurons, and thus compensate for mitochondrial dysfunction." They concluded, "The results of this pilot study provide a basis for further investigation of the effects of coconut oil, or its constituents, on neuronal survival focusing on mechanisms that may be involved."

In another noteworthy clinical trial involving 152 patients with Alzheimer's disease significant improvements were observed in the patients 45 and 90 days after they were supplied with MCFAs from coconut oil. The results of this trial resulted in the U.S. Food and Drug Administration (FDA) approving a synthetic form of caprylic acid known as *caprylidene* (trade name Axona) to be marketed as a "medical food." Yet it is highly probable that the same or similar benefits can be obtained simply by supplementing with coconut oil itself, which is not only much more affordable and widely available, but also free from side effects that Axona is known to produce. The side effects can range from coughing, dizziness, and fatigue, to gastrointestinal problems and high blood pressure, among other risk factors.

A Remarkable Case History

One of the most impressive examples of how supplementation with coconut oil can improve brain function was recounted by Mary T. Newport, MD in her book *Alzheimer's Disease: What If There Was a Cure?* Dr. Newport is a neonatal physician specializing in the care of sick newborn babies and babies born prematurely. To help the development of these babies' brains, neonatal physicians and nurses often provide the babies with MCFAs, since these same types of fats are also found in nursing mothers' breast milk. MCFAs are also a component of infant formulas.

In 2004, Dr. Newport's husband, Steve, then is his early 50s, was diagnosed with Alzheimer's disease after exhibiting signs of cognitive problems that first surfaced a few years earlier. During that time, Steve had also been diagnosed with clinical depression. Following his diagnosis of AD, Steve was prescribed the Alzheimer's drug Aricept. A year later, he was also placed on the drug Namenda. Neither drug helped his condition to any significant degree and in truth Steve continued to get worse.

Speaking about Steve's condition in an interview, Dr. Newport stated, "By 2008, he was actually doing very poorly. He had an MRI that showed that there was quite a bit of atrophy of the brain, and specifically in the areas that are consistent with Alzheimer's disease. He was losing weight. He had lost about ten pounds over three weeks. I realized he wasn't able to fix meals for himself while I was working. Even though he said he had and he thought he had eaten, he hadn't eaten. Things were kind of getting pretty bleak."

Desperate to find something that might slow down the progression of her husband's mental decline, Dr. Newport continued to scour the medical literature and searched for clinical trials for new drugs that Steve might be a candidate for. As a result, she happened upon a press release touting the benefits of Axona, the drug I mentioned above.

The press release stated that the results of the studies carried out on Axona showed that it improved the memories of approximately half of the patients who used it. Intrigued because she knew none of the other Alzheimer's drugs could make similar claims, Dr. Newport went online to further research Axona and came across the drug's patent application. "It was a very lengthy application," she says. "I learned a lot about Alzheimer's while I was reading this."

What most caught her attention was that Axona was developed to address the brain's insulin deficiency and insulin resistance in Alzheimer's patients. The concept of "diabetes of the brain," or "type 3 diabetes," had first been proposed in scientific papers published in 2005, but Dr. Newport had not been familiar with it until three years later when she discovered the patent application. Her discovery led her to go back to studies first published in the 1960s that revealed how the brain could make use of ketones as an alternative to glucose in order to supply itself with energy. It was during this same decade that scientists first discovered that when medium chain fatty acids, also known as medium chain triglycerides, or MCT oils, are consumed they are quickly converted into ketones by the liver, and then taken up by the brain to be used as an energy source. Putting all of these facts together, Dr. Newport realized that Axona acted as a synthetic version of MCT oils, which she was already familiar with because of her work as a neonatal physician. What she did not realize, however, until she read the patent application for Axona, was that the MCT oils used in neonatal care and in infant formulas were extracted from coconut oil.

Later the same day that she was putting all of this together, Dr. Newport's husband was once again screened to determine his brain condition, with the hope that he might qualify to participate in a clinical study. His score was too low for him to do so, and he was then given another specific test for Alzheimer's which involved asking him to draw a clock. He was unable to do so, at which point the doctor told Dr. Newport that his condition was much worse than she had thought, bordering on severe Alzheimer's.

This result spurred Dr. Newport to consider giving her husband coconut oil. After buying a bottle of it at her local health food store, Dr. Newport added two tablespoons of coconut oil to her husband's oatmeal for breakfast the next day. Later that same day, he was scheduled for another medical evaluation, this time scoring two points higher than he had the day before. Though she had no idea if the coconut oil had contributed to her husband's improved score or not, Dr. Newport decided to continue giving him coconut oil each day. In addition to the two tablespoons that she added to his breakfast, she purchased coconut oil cookbooks and began cooking with coconut oil for the other meals she made for her husband each day.

In her book, Dr. Newport recounts how her husband began to show improvement almost "right away" once the addition of coconut oil to his foods began. He became more alert, had more energy, and became more talkative and less depressed. "He said it was like the light switch came back on the day he started coconut oil," Dr. Newport reports.

Over time, Dr. Newport also shifted her husband to a low-carbohydrate diet and increased his daily dose of coconut oil, as well. She also began to use coconut oil and soon noticed improvements in her own memory and overall health. Her sister also began using coconut oil and reported that it improved her mental focus.

Once Dr. Newport added coconut oil to her husband's daily diet, she reports that "He improved very significantly and steadily the first year and remained stable for two more years." Eventually, however, he suffered a head injury from a fall from which he never fully recovered and which led to him experiencing seizures in 2013. "In spite of this serious setback, I feel it was well worth the extra quality time that we had together as a family," Dr. Newport states. "He remained in our home with the help of our wonderful caregivers and had minimal further worsening over the next two years. I cannot help but think that ketones played an important role in all of this."

Steve passed away at the start of January, 2016.

Because of how much her husband benefited from the addition of coconut oil to his diet, as well as her own ongoing research into the benefits of coconut and other MCT oils, and the research that others are also conducting on coconut oil in relation to Alzheimer's, dementia, and other diseases of the brain, Dr. Newport writes, "[T]here is now at least hope for others who are at risk or in earlier stages of this horrible disease [Alzheimer's], and their families might actually win their fight."

Since the publication of her book, Dr. Newport has heard from hundreds of others who have started using coconut and other MCT oils for their loved ones suffering from Alzheimer's and other conditions, including Parkinson's disease, multiple sclerosis (MS) and even two cases of Lou Gehrig's disease (ALS), all of whom experienced a stabilization of their disease's progression after they began using coconut oil. While some people experience no noticeable results, "the vast majority has reported improvements in cognitive functions and overall quality of life," Dr. Newport reports.

While it cannot be said unequivocally that coconut oil was the reason for the cognitive improvements and overall better quality of life Dr. Newport's husband experienced, neither can coconut oil be discounted as being a primary contributing factor that led to these benefits. "Studies of ketone esters for Alzheimer's, Parkinson's, and other neurodegenerative diseases urgently need to be undertaken, but funding for mass production of the ester and clinical testing has not yet materialized," Dr. Newport notes. "For now, you can provide ketones to the brain as an alternative fuel by consuming foods that contain medium chain triglycerides to produce ketones. What do you have to lose?"

Indeed.

To find out more about Dr. Newport's ongoing research, you can visit her website, www.coconutketones.com.

CONCLUSION

As this chapter explains, coconuts, and especially coconut oil, can help improve and maintain the health or your brain and lower the risk of developing brain conditions, including Alzheimer's and dementia, because of how quickly they produce ketones in the body once they are consumed. Ketones not only act as an alternative fuel source for the brain, they can also help prevent the occurrence of insulin resistance within the brain and the onset of "type 3 diabetes," or "diabetes of the brain" that is a hallmark of Alzheimer's and dementia.

Coconuts and coconut oil by themselves are not "magic bullets" for maintaining and improving brain health, of course. Other factors, such as a low-carbohydrate diet (especially a ketogenic diet, which is low in carbohydrates and rich in high-quality healthy fats, such as the MCFAs coconuts contain, along with moderate amounts of high-quality proteins), adequate exercise, stress management, and healthy sleep, are also important. So, too, is a properly functioning immune system. Boosting immune function is another significant benefit that coconuts can provide. To find out how and why this is so turn to Chapter 6.

6.

Coconuts and Your Immune System

Your overall health depends on the health of your body's immune system. And in today's modern world your immune system is under assault like never before, which is why it is so important that you do everything you can to support it. In this chapter, you will learn why adding coconut and its milk and oil to your diet can help you do so. Let's begin by examining what your immune system actually is and what it does.

MEET YOUR IMMUNE SYSTEM

Your immune system is made up of a complex, interwoven network of organs, cells, and biochemical substances. Together they work to protect your body against a broad spectrum of harmful bacteria, viruses, fungi, and other microorganisms, as well as environmental toxins, that cause disease. All of us are exposed to such microorganisms and toxins on a daily basis. Your immune system is also responsible for eliminating damaged and dead cells in your body. In order to perform its many tasks efficiently it must remain healthy.

How Does Your Immune System Keep You Healthy?

There are three basic ways in which your immune system works to keep you healthy.

1. First, via your skin and gastrointestinal tract, both of which act as physical barriers to infectious agents, your immune system acts to prevent infectious microorganisms and toxins from taking hold inside your body.

2. But not all such infectious agents can always be prevented from entering your body. When they succeed in doing so your immune system employs its second line of defense, triggering an immune response that sends untold millions of specialized immune cells streaming through your bloodstream to engulf and/or kill off these germs and toxins, and to prevent them from spreading further and deeper into your body. During this second line of defense an inflammatory response can also occur, causing your body to warm, such as during fever, and/or for the affected areas of your body to redden or swell until your immune cells eliminate the harmful invaders.

3. If necessary, your immune system will move into a third stage response in which it calls upon various organs in your body, especially your liver, spleen and lymph nodes, to assist it in its task of keeping you healthy.

What Makes Up Your Immune System?

Your immune system is composed of a complex network of organs and cells that safeguard the body from foreign invaders, such as bacteria, viruses, and other harmful microorganisms that may trigger infections.

Organs and Organ systems

For the most part your immune system is made up of the following organs and organ systems:

Bone marrow. Your bone marrow produces the stem cells that eventually develop into the various types of immune cells needed to protect you from harmful microorganisms.

Liver. Your liver serves as your body's main filtering and waste-processing plant, breaking down and eliminating dead cells and the waste products they accumulate, as well as helping to kill off harmful infectious agents in your bloodstream.

Lymphatic system. Your lymphatic system acts as your body's master drainage system. Your lymphatic system is made up of groups of immune tissue called lymph nodes that detect and filter out harmful substances in the lymph fluid that flows throughout your body, helping to maintain and regulate the fluid level of your cells and carrying various substances from body tissues to the blood. The primary concentrations of lymph nodes are located in your neck, armpits, chest, groin, and abdomen. When infections take hold in your body, these parts of your body can become swollen until the infections are eliminated.

Pancreas. Your pancreas also secretes various enzymes to not only assist in the digestion of the foods you eat, but also to attack and eliminate foreign microoganisms. One such enzyme produced by your pancreas is called *chymotrypsin*. It is released directly into the bloodstream where it seeks out infectious agents, as well as diseased and dead cells in your body. Once chymotrypsin identifies such microorganisms and cells, it goes to work eating away their protective coating, a substance called fibrin. Fibrin serves to help unhealthy cells and infectious agents from being detected by immune cells. As fibrin is stripped away these various immune cells become better able to recognize and eliminate such cells and microorganisms.

Skin and mucous membranes. Your skin and mucous membranes work together to create a protective barrier to keep toxins and infectious microorganisms from penetrating inside your body.

Spleen. Your spleen is home to the immune cells that manufacture antibodies, as well as immune cells known as lymphocytes and macrophage cells. Your spleen also acts as a filteear in your body, keeping it healthy and resistant to infections.

Stomach and gastrointestinal tract. Your stomach and gastrointestinal tract secretes stomach acid and enzymes to destroy and eliminate harmful invaders before they can pass from the GI tract into your bloodstream.

Thymus gland. Your thymus gland produces thymosin, a hormone that strengthens your body's immune response and helps regulate the functions of immune-boosting cells known as lymphocytes.

Immune Cells

In addition to these organs and organ systems, your immune system is also made up of various immune cells. These include lymphocytes, which produce antibodies, as well as B cell, T cells, and natural killer (NK) cells, macrophages, and neutrophils, as well as the immune boosting proteins interferon and interleukin.

Interferon. Interferon is a type of protein produced by your body in response to invading infectious agents, especially viruses. Interferon also helps to regulate your body's immune response to help prevent autoimmune reactions. Today, a number of interferon drugs modeled on the natural interferon your body produces are used to treat various health conditions, including autoimmune diseases, such as multiple sclerosis (MS), hepatitis B and C, and certain types of cancer and leukemia.

Interleukin. Another type of protein that plays an important role within your body's immune system is interleukin. It acts as a messenger, or signaling protein, and helps to trigger the activation of T cells. It also helps to regulate the overall function of lymphocytes. As with interferon, natural interleukin has also been modeled to create interleukin drugs, which are primarily used in the treatment of certain types of cancer.

Lymphocytes. Lymphocytes are a special class of white blood cells. Depending on the person, they make up between 25 to 40 percent of one's total blood cell count. There is an average of one trillion lymphocytes in the adult human body, and, combined, they produce approximately 100 trillion antibodies. Also known as immunoglobulins, antibodies are Y-shaped proteins produced from B cells as part of your body's immune response to invading bacteria, viruses, and other harmful microorganisms. Lymphocytes are produced in your body's bone marrow and increase in number when infections arise, as well as in response to diseases, such as cancer. They are primarily concentrated in lymph nodes, the spleen, and the thymus gland.

As mentioned, B cells, T cells, and natural killer (NK) cells are also produced by lymphocytes.

- **B cells** are formed within the lymph nodes of the lymphatic system, where they mature until they are needed to go to work against infectious agents. B cells secrete antibodies that can neutralize harmful microorganisms, as well as dying and dead cells.

- **T cells** are concentrated in the thymus gland (hence their name). They, too, react to and attempt to eliminate infectious microorganisms, as well as cancer cells. There are two primary classes of T cells, helper T cells (also called T4 or CD4 cells) and suppressor T cells.

  Helper T cells secrete immune boosting proteins, especially interferon and interleukin to stimulate B cells and macrophages. They also activate NK cells.

  Suppressor T cells, on the other hand, help to regulate the activity of your body's antibodies to prevent excessive immune reactions, which, if left unchecked, can result in the body literally attacking itself, which is what happens when autoimmune conditions take hold in the body.

- **Natural killer (NK) cells,** as their name implies, work to quickly kill and eliminate any foreign invading microorganism as soon as such organisms make contact within your body. They are also tasked with destroying dead and cancerous cells. In order to do this, NK cells act as your immune system's free-ranging surveillance system, and carry out their tasks by producing approximately 100 biochemical substances capable of destroying foreign cells and invaders.

Macrophages. Macrophages are another class of white blood cell. They serve your body's immune system by engulfing invading microorganisms and other foreign substances and then releasing enzymes to destroy them. By and large, macrophages ingest, or "vacuum up" anything inside your body that is not supposed to be there, including not only foreign invaders but also old, dying, and dead blood cells.

Neutrophils. Neutrophils are colorless blood cells that are also formed in the bone marrow. They, too, are released into the bloodstream at the first sign of invading microorganisms, especially harmful bacteria and fungi. Like microphages, their primary function is to ingest and then destroy such foreign invaders.

Risk Factors That Cause Your Immune System To Weaken

When your immune system is healthy and functioning optimally, its marvelous network of organs, immune cells, and the biochemical substances the immune cells release all work together to fend off and protect you from otherwise harmful microorganisms and toxins, without you even being aware of its actions. It is only when your immune system becomes compromised that exposure to invading infectious agents and toxins are able to establish footholds on or in your body and push you down the pathway of disease.

Although it is commonly believed that immune function starts to decline as we grow older, in actuality age-related decline in immunity is by no means inevitable. Most often it is not age but a variety of other factors that result in impaired immune function, and thus the development of the various types of diseases that the immune system is designed to prevent and protect against.

Two of the most common factors that can cause your immune system to weaken are poor diet and a lack of the nutrients that your immune system depends upon to function properly. By adding coconuts and coconut oil to your daily diet, you can go a long way towards improving your diet and maintaining your body's nutritional status.

HOW COCONUTS CAN BOOST IMMUNE FUNCTION

Many of the nutrients that coconuts and coconut oil contain (*see* Chapter 2) support immune function and are known to protect against harmful microorganisms. But the primary reason that coconuts and its oil can be so effective in boosting immunity and safeguarding against infectious diseases lies in the rich supply of medium-chain fatty acids (MCFAs) that they contain.

MCFA Fatty Acids

When coconuts or coconut oils are consumed, these MCFAs are quickly metabolized in the body, where they not only go to work to protect the heart and the brain, as you learned about in chapters 4 and 5 but also to be transformed into potent antimicrobials capable of fighting off unhealthy bacteria, viruses, fungi, and parasites.

Many of these harmful microorganisms possess an exterior membrane that is made up of fats (lipids). These fatty membranes are highly fluid and flexible, enabling the microorganisms to bend and squeeze their way inside your body's cells, tissues, and organs to trigger disease. Examples of bacteria that possess a lipid membrane include chlamydia, *H. pylori,* listeria, staphylococcus, and bacteria in the streptococcus family. Lipid-coated viruses include cytomegalovirus, Epstein-Barr, hepatitis C, herpes viruses, HIV, influenza (flu) viruses, measles virus, and pathogens in the orthopneumovirus family, which can cause pneumonia and other diseases of the respiratory tract.

Because the MCFAs coconuts contain are similar to the lipids that coat such bacteria and viruses, they attract themselves to these microorganisms to be absorbed within them. Once inside them, the MCFAs go to work to weaken the microorganisms' lipid coating, causing it to break apart and rupture. This, in turn, causes the microorganisms to die, with their remnants being mopped up and eliminated by the body's immune cells. Unlike pharmaceutical antibiotics and antiviral drugs, coconut's MCFAs accomplish this without damaging healthy cells, tissues, and organs, making them an optimal choice for protecting against such infectious agents. In addition, applying coconut oil topically can enhance the immune-protecting properties of your skin, adding further protection against skin conditions caused by infections.

Lauric Acid

When it comes to preventing and killing off bacterial and viral infections, lauric acid, one of the primary fatty acids of the MCFAs that coconuts and coconut oil contain, plays a major role. Lauric acid has been known to be a potent protective aid against infections by traditional healing cultures around the world for centuries, including in Mediterranean countries, such as France, Greece, Italy, and Morocco, where it is found in the fruits and seeds of the bay laurel tree native to those countries. Here in the United States, scientists first began to study lauric acid's healing properties beginning in the 1950s, primarily using coconut oil and palm kernel oil, since they have the highest concentrations of this medium-chain fatty acid.

Monolaurin

What researchers have discovered is that lauric acid is transformed into a substance called monolaurin once it is consumed and metabolized in the body. Monolaurin was first discovered by Jon J. Kabara, PhD, Professor Emeritus of Chemistry and Pharmacology at Michigan State University, who called it "one of the most exceptional and inspiring fats found in nature." His research found that monolaurin derived from coconuts is very deadly to invading bacteria and viruses, so much so that it is now marketed as an antibacterial and antiviral supplement under the brand name Lauricidin, a product developed by Dr. Kabara and his associates. But you can obtain the same benefits that Lauricidin provides by consuming coconuts and coconut oil. Moreover, unlike Lauricidin supplements, coconuts and coconut oil contain a variety of co-factor ingredients that enhance the body's ability to make better use of all of the MCFAs that coconut and its oil contain.

Mother's Milk

To anyone familiar with the care of newborn babies and infant development, the powerful benefits the MCFAs of coconuts have to boost immune function will not be surprising, since coconut's MCFAs are very similar to the medium-chain fatty acids contained in human breast milk. Mothers' milk not only nourishes babies, it also protects them from infectious disease in much the same way that coconut's MCFAs do. This is vitally important for the newborns' survival since their immune system is not yet fully developed. It is for this same reason that MCFAs are a primary ingredient in baby formulas—they too help keep babies healthy and the MCFAs the formulas contain are often derived from coconuts and coconut oil.

As I mentioned above, the MCFAs in coconuts and coconut oil are also highly effective in protecting against and eliminating fungi. One of the most common fungal infections in the U.S. today is candidiasis, also known as candidia, which is caused by the fungus *Candida albicans,* a single-celled, yeast-like fungus that naturally occurs in the body's gastrointestinal tract, where it helps the body to absorb and metabolize B vitamins.

Candidiasis

Under normal conditions, *C. albicans* is kept in check by the naturally-occurring healthy bacteria and other intestinal flora that are also found in the GI tract. Due to factors such as poor diet, excess sugar intake, nutritional deficiencies, the use of birth control drugs, and the overuse of antibiotics, however, these healthy bacteria and flora can become overwhelmed or killed off, causing the body's mechanisms for keeping *C. albicans* in check to be disrupted. When this happens it allows for the rampant spread of the fungus throughout the GI tract and into the bloodstream.

Candidiasis can manifest in the mouth as oral thrush, or systemically as yeast overgrowth affecting the entire body and resulting in a wide range of symptoms, including headache, gastrointestinal disorders, chronic fatigue, depression, mood swings, muscle pain, allergies, sinus infections, low immune function, and impaired cognitive function. In women, candidiasis can also occur as a vaginal yeast infection.

The treatment of candidiasis can often prove challenging and can take time. The most successful treatment approaches incorporate several of the basic principles of holistic medicine, which emphasizes self-care, proper diet, and the wise use of both conventional and complementary therapies. Since a variety of factors are usually responsible for candidiasis, each of them needs to be addressed directly. Because candidiasis usually results from these factors occurring over a prolonged period of time, patients must realize that there is no quick-fix cure. In order to be effective, both time and personal commitment to dietary and lifestyle changes are required.

Proper treatment also depends on the degree of yeast overgrowth and how badly it has compromised immune function. When yeast overgrowth is confined only to the gastrointestinal (GI) tract or vagina, the treatment tends to be shorter and less involved. In systemic cases, however, where yeast toxins have spread throughout the body, treatment protocols can last as long as six months to a year. And in severe cases of leaky gut syndrome, successful treatment (requiring the healing of the bowel lining) takes at least a year or more.

Many holistic physicians prescribe a four-stage approach in treating systemic candidiasis. The four stages consist of:

1. Killing the yeast overgrowth

2. Eliminating the fuel for the growth of candida through a yeast-free diet

3. Restoring normal friendly bacteria in the bowel

4. Strengthening the immune system

In the first stage of treatment the use of antifungal drugs such as Nystatin or Diflucan are often employed. While such drugs can be effective in killing the *C. albicans* fungus, they can also cause a variety of unpleasant side effects and can take a toll on the liver. Fortunately, research has found that caprylic acid, one of the MCFAs contained in coconuts and coconut oil, is also highly effective in killing of *C. albicans* without the risks of side effects that antifungal drugs pose. Because of this research, caprylic acid supplements derived from coconuts and its oil are now marketed and sold in health food stores as a remedy for candidiasis, as well as for other types of fungal infections. But people who suffer from candidiasis and other fungal infections can get the same results simply by using coconut oil instead. The antifungal properties of caprylic acid found in coconuts and coconut oil is further bolstered by the lauric acid they contain, which, once it is converted into monolaurin, also has antifungal properties.

Applying coconut oil topically can often prove effective for treating fungal infections on the skin and nails, as well. And by adding coconuts and coconut oil to your daily diet you can significantly reduce your risk of developing candidiasis and other types of fungal infections in the first place. This fact is demonstrated by the cultures around the world where coconut and its oil are dietary staples. In such cultures, such fungal infections are extremely rare.

The reason why this is so can be found in a research study performed by scientists at the Department of Medical Microbiology and Parasitology at University College Hospital in Ibadan, Nigeria. About the study, which was published in 2007 in the *Journal of Medicinal Food*, the scientists wrote, "The emergence of antimicrobial resistance, coupled with the availability of fewer antifungal agents with fungicidal actions, prompted this present study to characterize Candida species in our environment and determine the effectiveness of virgin coconut oil as an antifungal agent on these species." In the study, the scientists exposed 52 isolates of *Candida* species to coconut oil. Of these forms, *C. albicans,* was found to have the highest susceptibility to coconut oil, which killed the *C. albicans* strain 100 percent of the time. Based on their findings, the scientists recommended that, "Coconut oil should be used in the treatment of fungal infections in view of emerging drug-resistant Candida species."

Parasite Infections

The addition of coconuts and coconut oil to your daily diet can also protect you against infections caused by food and water borne parasites. There are two main classes of parasites, worms (for example, roundworms and tapeworms) and protozoa, such as cryptosporidium and giardia. Parasite infections are commonly thought to only be problems in Third World countries where poor sanitation is widespread. In reality, however, both classes of parasites are far more prevalent in the United States than most people realize.

Protozoa, which, like *C. albicans,* are single-celled organisms widely found in our nation's lakes, rivers, and streams that provide approximately 50 percent of all U.S. tap water. Though municipal tap water is treated before it is made available to the public for drinking and other uses, such treatment methods do not always succeed in killing off protozoa, especially in smaller municipalities. This is particularly true of giardia, the cause of the most common type of parasite infection (known as giardiasis) found in the

U.S. According to the Centers for Disease Control and Prevention (CDC), giardiasis affects an estimated two million Americans each and every year as a result of them drinking contaminated water.

Like many bacteria and viruses, giardia has a protective coating that surrounds it, making it possible to sometimes resist being killed off by water treatment facilities. The MCFAs in coconuts and coconut oil are capable of penetrating and destroying this protective coating, just as they do to lipid-coated bacteria and viruses. Because of this, adding coconuts and coconut oil to your daily diet can help protect you from such parasite infections. Doing so is an especially good idea if you live in an area in which outbreaks of giardiasis have already occurred.

Both coconut oil and the dried meat of coconuts have long been used by healers in the lands in which coconuts grow to also protect against parasitic worms, both those that can infect the GI tract, and topical worms, such as head lice. In Ayurveda, the century's oldest system of medicine in India and other parts of southeastern Asia, for example, both coconut oil and dried coconut meat are prescribed to expel intestinal worms, while the topical application of coconut oil is known to be a proven Ayurvedic remedy for treating and preventing head lice.

Based on what you have read in this section, I trust you now have a better understanding of how and why the addition of coconuts and coconut oil to your diet can help maintain and improve your body's immune system by helping it resist the ongoing assault it faces by infectious bacteria, viruses, fungi, and even parasites. Not only is coconut delicious, in a very real sense it and its oil also act a powerful medicinal food, even against one of today's most feared viruses.

NEW HOPE FOR PEOPLE WITH HIV

One of the most impressive and important findings about the immune-enhancing benefits of coconuts and coconut oil in recent years has to do with HIV (human immunodeficiency virus) which is believed to cause AIDS.

The first researcher to publish clinical studies about the benefits that coconut oil can provide for HIV and AIDS patients was the late Conrado S. Dayrit, MD (May 31, 1919 to October 5, 2007), who was Professor Emeritus of Pharmacology at the University of the Philippines College of Medicine and cofounder and past president of the Philippine Heart Association. Because of how extensively Dr. Dayrit studied the medicinal properties of coconuts and coconut oil, he was dubbed "Dr. Coconut." He referred to virgin coconut oil as "a drugstore in a bottle" due to the many health benefits his research confirmed coconut oil provides.

Dr. Dayrit's pioneering research on the use of coconut oil to treat HIV and AIDS was triggered by the research dating back to the 1970s conducted by Dr. Kabara and others that revealed the antimicrobial properties of the MCFAs in coconut and its oil, as well as a 1997 presentation by noted health researcher, the late Mary G. Enig, PhD (July 13, 1931 to September 8, 2014) at a symposium in the Philippines. In her presentation, Dr. Enig shared that the AIDS organization, Keep Hope Alive, had documented that coconut oil, either taken separately, or in conjunction with anti-HIV medications that had previously not been effective, had reduced the viral load of a number of patients with HIV or full blown AIDs, in some cases to levels that were undetectable. "The amount of coconut oil consumed (50 ml or 3 1/2 table-spoonfuls) or half of a coconut, would contain 20 to 25 grams of lauric acid, which indicates that the oil is metabolized in the body to release lauric acid and/or monolaurin," Dr. Dayrit wrote.

In 1999, Dr. Dayrit conducted his own study with HIV patients, using either monolaurin or virgin coconut oil to treat them. There were 15 partici-pants in the study, five men and ten women, ranging in age between 22 and 38 years old. All of the patients were too poor to be able to afford medication for HIV/AIDS, nor had they ever received medication prior to the start of the study. They were treated by Dr. Dayrit at San Lazaro Hospital, a facility for infectious diseases located in Manila, Philippines.

At the beginning of the study, seven of the patients were found to have elevated liver enzymes, two of them had high cholesterol levels, and one had elevated levels of triglycerides. Twelve patients also presented with unex-plained eosinophilia, a condition characterized by higher than normal white blood cell (eosinophils) levels, and one of the patients suffered from renal (kidney) dysfunction. "Their viral load ranged from 1,960 to 1,190,000 except for one patient whose load was too low to count (below 400)," Dr. Dayrit reported.

The patients were randomly assigned to three treatment groups. In the first group, patients received high doses of monolaurin daily, administered three times each. The second group received a low daily dose of monolaurin, also administered three times a day. "The monolaurin used was 95 percent pure, "Dr. Dayrit wrote. The third group received three daily doses of extra virgin coconut oil equivalent to the amount of monolaurin received by the first group (approximately three and a half tablespoons per day).

The patients in all three groups were monitored daily to screen for any potential side effects caused by their treatment. In addition, at the begin-ning of the study, which lasted for six months, the patients were adminis-tered blood tests, which were repeated three months later, and in the sixth month, following the end of their treatment. The tests included monitoring the patients' body weight, testing of the patient's viral load using the PCR method, assessment of their CD4 and CD8 immune cells counts, complete blood count (CBC), liver function tests, kidney function tests, and tests of their HDL, LDL, total cholesterol, and triglycerides levels. According to Dr. Dayrit, treatment benefit was defined as a reduction in the patients' viral load and an increase in their CD4 count.

On the third month of the study, the patient who originally presented with an undetectable viral load was shown to still have an undeterminable viral load and was therefore excluded from the study's computations. Of the remaining 14 patients, a total of seven patients from all three groups had achieved a decreased viral load count (two in the high monolaurin group, two in the low monolaurin group, and three in the group that received extra virgin coconut oil). The remaining seven patients all exhibited an increased viral load. By month six, the viral load had decreased in a total of eight patients across all three groups, with the most significant decreases occurring in two patients who received coconut oil and one in the low monolaurin group. A total of 11 patients also gained weight (weight gain ranged from slightly over two pounds to just over 50 pounds), and five patients also showed a positive increase in their CD4 and CD8 counts. None of the patients in the study experienced any serious side effects from their treatment.

Three patients developed AIDS in the third month of therapy when their CD4 count dropped below 200. One of these three, who was in the coconut oil group, died two weeks after the study was completed. The two other AIDS patients were in the low monolaurin group. One of them fully recovered by month six, while the other patient showed "a rapid return towards normal CD4 and CD8 counts." Two of these significant decreases were in the coconut oil group and one in the low monolaurin group. The two patients were also among the 11 who experienced positive weight gain over the course of the study.

"This initial trial confirmed the anecdotal reports that coconut oil does have an antiviral effect and can beneficially reduce the viral load of HIV patients," Dr. Dayrit wrote."The positive antiviral action was seen not only with the monoglyceride of lauric acid [monolaurin] but with coconut oil itself. This indicates that coconut oil is metabolized to monoglyceride forms of C-8, C-10, C-12 [monoloaurin] to which it must owe its anti-pathogenic activity. More and longer therapies using monolaurin will have to be designed and done before the definitive role of such coconut products can be determined. With such products, the outlook for more efficacious and cheaper anti HIV therapy is improved."

Like many other viruses, HIV has a lipid (fat) coating. Whereas HIV and AIDS drugs work by attacking the genetic material with the HIV virus, they can also cause a range of potentially serious side effects. By contrast, as you learned above, the lauric acid and other MCFAs contained in coconut oil work by weakening and dissolving the lipid coating of the HIV virus, causing it to be destroyed. Moreover, they do so without the risk of serious side effects. In addition, coconut oil costs a fraction of what HIV and AIDS drugs cost.

While it would be irresponsible to claim that coconut oil is a cure for HIV and AIDS—no study has established that it is—the research by Dr. Dayrit and others has conclusively shown that coconut oil *can* help to relieve some of the symptoms of HIV/AIDS, and in some cases also boost the immune systems of HIV/AIDS patients. This research also adds to the growing body of research that shows that coconut oil, as well as coconuts themselves, do indeed have powerful immune boosting benefits that can be obtained simply by adding coconuts and coconut oil to your daily diet.

CONCLUSION

Given the powerful benefits that coconuts and coconut oil provide for the health of the immune system, now that you've read this chapter I hope you have a better understanding as to why adding coconuts and coconut oil to your diet can go a long way to keeping your immune system functioning optimally. Neither coconuts nor coconut oil of themselves are "magic bullets" when it comes to boosting immunity, of course. To most properly care for your immune system, and therefore your overall health, you also need to eat healthy, drink a plentiful supply of pure filtered water each day to keep your body hydrated, get regular exercise, manage your stress, and get adequate amounts of deep, restful sleep. Hopefully, you are already taking such measures. Adding coconuts and coconut oil to your daily diet will serve to enhance these measures, making you further resistant to infectious disease.

Now that you've learned about how coconut and its oil can improve immune function, let's examine the benefits they have for maintaining healthy blood pressure. That is the topic of Chapter 7, *Coconuts and High Blood Pressure.*

7.

Coconuts and
High Blood Pressure

High blood pressure, or hypertension, is a serious health condition that can lead to other health problems, including heart attack and stroke. According to the American Heart Association, approximately one-third of all American adults have high blood pressure, including many people in their early 20s, and another third of all American suffer from pre-hypertension, meaning their blood pressure levels are higher than normal. In addition, all too often high blood pressure is also undiagnosed. Over 20 percent of people with high blood pressure are not aware of their condition. For this reason, high blood pressure is often referred to as "the silent killer" because the damage it can cause within the body can go undetected until it is too late to prevent heart attack, stroke, and other conditions that high blood pressure can cause.

Although high blood pressure is not a disease, per se, it is a valuable marker for heart disease, and therefore it is important that it be monitored. Blood pressure readings of 120/80 mmHg are considered normal. The number 120 is called the systolic blood pressure, which is the pressure in the artery when the heart pumps. The number 80 is called the diastolic blood pressure, which is the pressure in the artery when the heart relaxes (fills). Each blood pressure increase of 20/10 mmHg can double the risk of heart disease. Before age 50, the diastolic blood pressure is the best predictor of heart disease risk; after age 50, the systolic blood pressure is a better indicator of risk.

When measuring blood pressure, it is best to use arm cuffs, not wrist or finger monitors. If your doctor finds that your blood pressure is high, he or she may recommend blood pressure medication. In cases of dangerously high blood pressure levels, such drugs can literally be lifesavers. However, although such drugs may relieve the symptoms of high blood pressure, they do little or nothing to resolve its underlying causes. Additionally, many of these drugs can cause unhealthy side effects. Therefore, if you have high blood pressure, ask your doctor to help you determine whatever factors may be contributing to your condition.

UNDERSTANDING HIGH BLOOD PRESSURE

The term *blood pressure* is used to describe the force of blood against the walls of your body's blood vessels (veins and arteries) and the chambers of the heart itself. High blood pressure occurs whenever blood vessels anywhere in your body, primarily the arteries and smaller arteries known as arterioles, become constricted. Such constriction can be temporary or become chronic, depending on the causative factors involved. For example, under times of stress or anger blood vessels constrict, causing blood pressure levels to rise, but usually they will relax again and blood pressure will subside back to normal once anger or the stressful situation passes. However, chronic stress, anger, and other factors, such as atherosclerosis (hardening of the arteries), can lead to ongoing arterial constriction and thus chronically high blood pressure levels.

Whether fleeting or ongoing, whenever constriction occurs your body's blood vessels increase their resistance to the flow of blood throughout your body. This, in turn, forces your heart to work harder to move blood through your blood vessels to deliver the oxygen and nutrients your blood supplies to your cells, tissues, and organs. If high blood pressure becomes chronic, the additional energy and effort required by your heart to keep blood flowing properly throughout your body can take a toll on your heart muscles.

This causes a multitude of serious problems, such as damage to heart muscles, as well as increasing the risk of heart attack, stroke, and other cardiovascular disease, including congestive heart failure. In addition, prolonged periods of high blood pressure can impair kidney function and lead to kidney failure, as well as circulation problems in the body, especially the lower extremities, and also increase the risk of premature death. The damage caused by prolonged high blood pressure can also make it easier for toxins, oxidized cholesterol, and harmful bacteria to take hold and form dangerous deposits on the artery walls. This further increases the risk of premature death and/or the onset of the above mentioned diseases.

Types of High Blood Pressure

There are two types of high blood pressure. The first and by far the most common type is known as essential hypertension and refers to high blood pressure for which doctors are unable to determine a specific underlying cause. Over 90 percent of all cases of high blood pressure are essential hypertension.

The second type of high blood pressure is known as secondary hypertension. As its name implies, this type of high blood pressure is the result, or a secondary factor, of a previously existing health condition. It usually results from kidney disease or malfunction or impaired functioning of one or more organs in your body's endocrine (hormone) system.

Symptoms of High Blood Pressure

The reason high blood pressure so often goes undetected is because it often presents no obvious symptoms. In addition, when symptoms are present, they are often misconstrued as health problems not related to blood pressure. Such symptoms can include:

- dizziness

- fatigue

- feelings of restlessness or irritability

- headache

- sleeping problems, such as insomnia

Gastrointestinal problems, as well as difficulty breathing and other respiratory problems, can also be symptoms of high blood pressure. If you suffer from such problems it is important that you consult with a physician, especially if the problems persist.

Cause of High Blood Pressure

In addition to chronic stress and upsetting emotions, a variety of other factors can cause the most common type of high blood pressure (essential hypertension). They include:

- excess consumption of alcohol, coffee, and other caffeinated drinks

- exposure to environmental toxins (especially heavy metals, such as lead or mercury)

- insufficient consumption of water each day (chronic low-grade dehydration)

- lack of regular restful sleep

- poor diet and nutritional deficiencies

- unhealthy dietary fats

- unhealthy lifestyle choices, such as smoking and lack of exercise

Many pharmaceutical drugs can also cause blood pressure levels to spike and remain elevated, as can feelings of loneliness, anxiety, and depression caused by social isolation.

COCONUTS CAN HELP KEEP YOUR BLOOD PRESSURE LEVELS HEALTHY

As you learned in Chapter 4, people in Polynesia and other regions of the world who follow a coconut-rich diet and use coconut oil for cooking and baking have a much lower incidence of heart disease than do people in the U.S. and other Western nations. Similarly, people in countries in which coconuts and coconut oil are dietary staples also have a low incidence of high blood pressure. Research indicates that one reason this is so is because of the anti-inflammatory effects the saturated, medium-chain fatty acids (MCFAs) found in coconuts and coconut oil have in the body once they are consumed.

Omega-6 Fatty-acids Can Raise Blood Pressure Levels

As it does in many other health conditions, including heart disease and atherosclerosis, chronic inflammation plays a significant role in the onset and perpetuation of high blood pressure. In Chapter 3, you learned that many unsaturated fats, particularly those high in omega-6 fatty acids, can cause inflammation. Because they do so, their addition in food products and their use for cooking and baking can be a major contributing factor in the development of high blood pressure. By contrast, the MCFAs in coconut and its oil have the opposite effect and are capable of reducing inflammation levels in the body, as well as oxidative stress, which is another cause of high blood pressure.

One of the reasons the excessive use of omega-6 fatty acids can increase blood pressure levels and increase health risks overall has to do with what happens when they are consumed. In addition to increasing levels of oxidative stress in the body, they are converted into substances called prostaglandins.

Prostaglandin

Some prostaglandins, such as those produced from omega-3 fatty acids, have beneficial effects in the body, including reducing inflammation and helping to maintain healthy blood vessels. An overabundance of prostaglandins derived from omega-6 fatty acids, however, can be detrimental to your health. Research has shown that they can increase inflammation levels in the body and cause blood vessels to constrict. They can also increase platelet stickiness.

Platelets

Platelets, also called *thrombocytes,* are cell-like particles in the blood that help the normal blood clotting process that occurs in response to cuts and bleeding. When such incidents occur, platelets clump, or stick, together to form a plug or seal on blood vessels, while also releasing chemicals that further aid in the clotting process. Under normal conditions, this platelet response ends when healing occurs. Ongoing platelet stickiness, however, can cause blood to clot excessively, causing blood vessels to constrict and blood pressure levels to rise, while also increasing the risk of atherosclerosis, heart attack, and stroke.

MCFAs and Exercise to Lower Blood Pressure

Unlike either omega-3 or omega-6 fatty acids, the MCFAs in coconuts and coconut oil do not get converted into prostaglandins. In addition, when coconut oil is used for cooking and baking its MCFAs are not oxidized, as all omega-3 and 6 fatty acids are when they are exposed to heat. Just as importantly, the inclusion of coconuts and coconut oil to your diet can reduce the effects of excessive, harmful prostaglandins in the body, thus reducing inflammation and, therefore, the risk of high blood pressure, as well as many other conditions.

Lauric Acid

Animal studies have determined that the MCFA lauric acid, one of the primary fatty acids in coconuts, has an especially positive effect in reducing inflammation and oxidative stress associated with high blood pressure. In one recent study, researchers studied the effects of lauric acid derived from coconut oil on both normal and hypertensive rats. They found that the administration of lauric acid to both rat populations successfully reduced blood pressure levels in both groups. Moreover, their research showed that lauric acid also reduced oxidative stress in the rats' hearts and kidneys, and triggered a release of constriction (vasorelaxation) in the rats' arteries. They also found that lauric acid acted as an overall antioxidant, which is also significant, since antioxidants help to prevent and counteract free radical damage that can cause inflammation and is another risk factor for high blood pressure.

Baroflex

The study above builds on previous animal studies that have also demonstrated the benefits of using coconuts to lower high blood pressure. In another such study, researchers found that regular consumption of coconut oil along with regular exercise completely reversed high blood pressure in rats within five weeks.

In this study, the researchers keyed in on a primary mechanism in the body that regulates blood pressure levels, known as the baroreflex, or the baroreceptor reflex. This reflex helps to control blood pressure levels by sending nerve impulses from sensory nerve endings called baroreceptor sites that are located within the body's major arteries, including the aorta and the carotid arteries. These sites are highly sensitive to changes in blood pressure, and send signals to the brain that cause blood vessels to dilate (expand) and heart rate to decrease when blood pressure levels rise, and that causes constriction of blood vessels and an increased heart rate when blood pressure levels fall below normal. It is this process that helps the body to keep blood pressure levels under control.

The researchers who conducted this study first tested the rats' baroreflex sensitivity in order to assess how effectively it was functioning. Then, over the course of the five weeks, the rats were divided into four groups. One group was given coconut oil alone without exercise; another group exercised each day by swimming but did not receive coconut oil; a third group was given both coconut oil and swam daily; and the last group was sedentary and was fed a saline solution.

At the end of the five-week period, all but the sedentary rat group showed a reduction in their blood pressure levels, with the group that both exercised and received coconut oil showing the most impressive reduction in blood pressure. Testing of the rats' baroreflex at the end of the study period also revealed that the rats who received coconut oil and/or exercise had reduced baroreflex sensitivity, meaning they were able to maintain their blood pressure levels to a much greater degree than the sedentary rats.

An equally important finding from this study showed that both coconut oil and exercise reduced oxidative stress in the non-sedentary rats. The mice that did not receive coconut oil or exercise exhibited much greater oxidative stress, and the muscles of their hearts were forced to work harder. In addition, the researchers found that coconut oil and exercise had positive antioxidant effects on the rats' heart, aorta, and overall health of the rats' blood. Furthermore, the combination of coconut oil and exercise also reduced the rats' body weight.

"This [study] is an important finding as coconut oil is currently being considered a popular 'superfood' and it is being consumed by athletes and the general population who seek a healthy lifestyle," stated Dr. Valdir de Andrade Braga, a co-author of the study. "The possibility of using coconut oil as an adjuvant to treat hypertension adds to the long list of benefits associated with its consumption."

Human Studies

The ability of coconuts and coconut oil to help maintain healthy blood pressure levels has also been confirmed in a number of human studies. In one such study, two populations in Polynesia were examined. In the first group, 89 percent of their entire daily dietary fat consumption was obtained from coconut oil. In the other group, only seven percent of their dietary fat came from coconut oil, with the majority coming from other sources. The first group of Polynesians was found to have much healthier blood pressure levels overall compared to the second group.

Another study revealed two other important benefits of coconuts and coconut oil with regard to blood pressure. It is the Kitivan study that I first mentioned in Chapter 4, which is so named because it involved studying the dietary habits and health status of native people living in the Pacific island of Kitiva. In addition to finding that Kitivans who follow their traditional, coconut-rich diet have no incidence of heart disease or stroke, the study also found that the Kitivan people have virtually no incidence of high blood pressure, either. Yet their diet is high in saturated fats because of how rich it is in coconuts, coconut oil, and coconut water.

Two other significant findings also came out of this study. The first was that the Kitivan people's blood pressure levels remained healthy and did not increase to any significant degree as they grew older. By contrast, even among healthy people here in the West blood pressure levels typically do rise with age. Of even more significance, the Kitivans were also found to have low blood levels of insulin, meaning that they did not suffer from insulin resistance or insulin sensitivity, both of which are other risk factors that can cause blood pressure levels to rise. These two factors go a long way to explaining the Kitivans' excellent health status throughout their lives. You will learn more about the positive effects coconuts and coconut oil have on insulin in Chapter 8.

COCONUT WATER CAN ALSO HELP

Fresh coconut water has long been highly regarded as a healthy drink in all tropical cultures in which coconut trees grow. In Hawaii, for instance, coconut water is called *noelani*, which means "dew from the heavens" because of the refreshing benefits it provides. In recent decades, research has confirmed that fresh coconut water is indeed good for our health. Human studies have also found that coconut water from fresh young coconuts can help maintain healthy blood pressure levels both directly and indirectly.

One study involved 28 people with high blood pressure. For two weeks prior to any intervention, the study group's systolic and diastolic blood pressure levels were monitored daily. At the end of the two weeks, they were then divided into four groups. The first group served as the control group and its members were given bottled water to drink each day. The second group was given fresh coconut water to drink. The third group was given a beverage known as mauby, a traditional tropical drink made from buckthorn tree bark, and the third group was given combinations of coconut water and mauby to drink. No other interventions, either dietary or lifestyle-related, were implemented.

At the end of an additional two weeks, the systolic and diastolic blood pressure levels of the participants in all four groups were again tested. In the coconut water group, 71 percent of participants showed a significant decrease in their systolic blood pressure levels and 29 percent showed a marked decrease in their diastolic pressure. In the groups who drank either mauby or the combination of coconut water and mauby, 40 and 43 percent of the participants, respectively, also showed significant improvements in their blood pressure levels. By contrast, in the group who drank bottled water, 57 percent of the participants were found to have an increase in their systolic blood pressure levels, with no noticeable change in their diastolic levels.

As I mentioned above, chronic low-grade dehydration is another significant risk factor for high blood pressure. One of the ways we become dehydrated is by exercising or engaging in other types of physical activity. The importance of rehydrating after exercise has made so-called sports drinks increasingly popular in recent years. While such drinks can indeed rehydrate your body and restore nutrients and electrolytes that are lost during exercise, many sports drinks also contain unhealthy ingredients that can diminish their benefits. Research has shown that fresh coconut water is a healthier alternative.

In one such study, the effectiveness of plain water, sports drinks, fresh young coconut water, and sodium-enriched fresh young coconut water on rehydration were compared. In the study, researchers wanted to know how effectively each of these beverages work as rehydration agents and how well they restore overall plasma volume. (Plasma is a type of fluid found in both blood and lymph.)

The study involved ten healthy males who exercised for 90 minutes in a temperature-controlled environment to induce dehydration. As a result of this exercise the participants lost an average of three percent of their body weight in water. For two hours after the exercise period, the participants were given either plain water, a sports drink, fresh young coconut water, or sodium-enriched fresh young coconut water to drink. After the two hours it was found that the participants who drank either fresh young coconut water, a sports drink, or the sodium-enriched fresh young coconut water all experienced higher levels of rehydration than those who drank plain water. Plasma volume improved in all but the plain water group, as well. The highest levels of rehydration occurred in the groups who drank either the sports drink or sodium-enriched fresh young coconut water, with both beverages producing nearly equal results. However, compared to both the sports drink and plain water groups, those in the sodium-enriched fresh young coconut water group also experienced less nausea and stomach upset. "In conclusion," the authors of the study wrote, "ingesting SCW [sodium-enriched fresh coconut water] was as good as ingesting a commercial sports drink for whole body rehydration after exercise-induced dehydration but with better fluid tolerance."

(It's important to note that the coconut water used in these studies was derived from fresh young coconuts. These coconuts are unlike the riper, brown coconuts commonly found in grocery stores, although they too can often be found in both grocery and health food stores. Look in the stores' refrigerated section, as they are highly perishable. The coconut water they provide is fresh, raw, and rich in nutrients. Commercial bottled coconut water is much different and not as healthy to drink because its nutritional content is not as fresh and often further diminished in potency due to being processed and pasteurized.)

OTHER STEPS YOU CAN TAKE TO MANAGE YOUR BLOOD PRESSURE LEVELS

While the addition of coconuts and coconut oil to your diet can help to maintain healthy blood pressure, this step alone is of course not a complete solution. Here are some other simple yet powerful steps you can take to prevent high blood pressure from developing and to reduce it if it already has developed. If your blood pressure level isn't at a dangerous level, take a few months implementing these self-care measures. In many cases, they can be enough to bring your blood pressure into a healthy range.

> **Note:** According to Michael Galitzer, MD, a leading integrative physician in Los Angeles, California, should you still require blood pressure medications after implementing these measures for a few months, you should take your medications at night. "Doing so will increase the medications' effectiveness by 25 to 50 percent, at the same dose, compared to when they are taken during the day," Dr. Galitzer says. "The only class of blood pressure medication for which this is not true is diuretic medication."

See Your Doctor and Get Tested

The first step is to consult with your doctor and have him or her measure your blood pressure. Doing so is a quick and easy procedure. Today, you can also find blood pressure monitors at your local drug store. Most of these devices are inexpensive and reasonably accurate, allowing you to check your blood pressure level on a regular basis without the need to see your doctor. However, if you currently do not know your blood pressure level, see your doctor so that he or she can work with you to create an optimal healthy lifestyle.

Diet

A healthy diet is one of the most important factors in preventing and reducing high blood pressure. Such a diet is one that is low in unhealthy fats and sugar and rich in foods containing potassium, calcium, and magnesium. Fiber-rich foods are also important. Overall, try to eat meals that contain plentiful supplies of fresh, organic vegetables, along with free-range lean meats and poultry and wild caught fish. Try to also limit your intake of carbohydrate foods.

In at least one meal each day try to include garlic and/or onions, both of which have been shown to reduce both systolic and diastolic blood pressure levels. Also be sure to eliminate all refined and simple carbohydrate foods, processed foods, and sodas and other unhealthy beverages, while drinking lots of pure, filtered water throughout the day.

And don't be afraid to add salt to your diet. Contrary to what was accepted as medical wisdom for decades, researchers are now finding that a salt-restrictive diet for most people is not actually healthy. Our bodies require salt in order to function properly, including maintaining healthy blood pressure levels. The best forms of salt contain both iodine and trace minerals. Good choices are sea salt and Celtic salt.

Nutritional Supplements

There are a number of nutrients that can help keep blood pressure levels under control. Some of the most beneficial are vitamins B3 and B6 along with a complete B-complex supplement, vitamin C, omega-3 fatty acids, magnesium, potassium, selenium, and zinc. Many of these nutrients are contained in coconuts and coconut oil. (*See* Chapter 2)

Herbal Remedies

One of the best herbal remedies for preventing and reducing high blood pressure is hawthorne. Hawthorne is well known for its ability to strengthen and protect the cardiovascular system, so it's not surprising that it is beneficial for helping to manage blood pressure levels too. Other helpful herbs include celery seed extract, which acts as a natural calcium channel blocker and olive leaf extract, which acts as a natural inhibitor of angiotensin converting enzyme (ACE) which can harm blood vessels and cause them to constrict, thus increasing the risk of hypertension.

Lifestyle

A healthy lifestyle is another significant factor for maintaining healthy blood pressure levels. Healthy life style choices include limiting your daily alcohol and caffeine intake, as well as not smoking and avoiding exposure to second-hand smoke. If you are overweight, seek help so that you can get to within ten pounds or less of your ideal weight, as healthy weight loss can dramatically reduce high blood pressure.

Managing stress is also very important, as chronic stress is one of the primary causes of high blood pressure. Meditation can be particularly effective in this regard, so much so in fact that in 1984 the National Institutes of Health (NIH) recommended meditation over prescription drugs as a treatment for mild cases of high blood pressure.

Regular exercise is also important. Exercise not only helps to lower high blood pressure, it is also excellent for reducing stress. One of the easiest and most enjoyable ways to obtain the benefits of exercise is to simply take a 20 to 30 minute walk once a day.

Social Health

In addition to the above steps, be honest with yourself and evaluate your relationships, both at work and at home. Try to avoid spending time with people who are habitually negative or who cause you stress in other ways. In addition, if you need help with your personal relationships, consider counseling or receiving some other type of guidance. Just as importantly, try not to spend too much time alone. Numerous scientific studies show that people with strong and supportive social ties on average are healthier, have better blood pressure levels, and usually live longer than people who tend to be "loners."

CONCLUSION

After reading this chapter I hope you have a better understanding of how and why maintaining healthy blood pressure is so important to your overall health. Please make it a point to monitor your blood pressure levels on a regular basis, especially if you know you have, or are at risk for developing, high blood pressure.

In this chapter, you also learned how and why coconuts, coconut oil, and the water from fresh, young coconuts can help improve and maintain blood pressure levels, giving you one more reason to consider adding them to your daily diet. Now, in Chapter 8, let's look at the ways in which coconuts and coconut oil can help you lose weight and address obesity, one of our nation's, and the world's, most serious health problems.

8.

Coconuts and Weight Loss

I t's a sad fact of life, both here in the United States and around the world: More and more people across the globe are not only overweight, they are obese. And that trend is increasing with each passing year.

According to the Centers for Disease Control and Prevention (CDC), throughout the 1980s not a single state in the U.S. had an obesity rate higher than 15 percent. Today, every state does, with 12 states having obesity rates of 30 percent or more. *All told, Americans are overweight by a collective 4.5 billion pounds.*

Two 2017 reports illustrate the severity of this problem. The first report comes from a published study in the *New England Journal of Medicine*, which states that 30 percent of the world's population—approximately 2.2 billion children and adults—today suffer from health conditions that are directly due to them being overweight or obese. According to the study's authors, that figure breaks down to nearly 108 million children and more than 600 million adults with a body mass index (BMI) greater than 30. (A BMI score of 30 is the threshold for obesity, whereas being overweight is defined as having a BMI score between 25 and 30. The BMI score is the measure of the percentage of a person's body fat in relation to their height and weight. It is calculated by dividing a person's weight, or mass, by the square of his or her height.)

The study, which examined the health status of more than 195 countries and territories between 1980 and 2015, found that the incidence of obesity in over 70 countries has doubled during that time span in more than 70 countries, and is continuously rising in most other nations of the world. Even more alarming, the study found that obesity in children is increasing at a greater rate than that of adults in many countries around the world. The highest level of obesity among children and young adults is occurring in the United States, with nearly 13 percent of that demographic now obese. This is the highest rate of childhood obesity among the world's 20 most populous nations.

LIFE-THREATENING CONDITIONS LINKED TO OBESITY

"Excess body weight is one of the most challenging public health problems of our time, affecting nearly one in every three people," states Dr. Ashkan Afshin, the paper's lead author and an Assistant Professor of Global Health at the Institute for Health Metrics and Evaluation (IHME).

"People who shrug off weight gain do so at their own risk—risk of cardiovascular disease, diabetes, cancer, and other life-threatening conditions," adds Dr. Christopher Murray, another author of the study and Director of IMHE at the University of Washington. "Those half-serious New Year's resolutions to lose weight should become year-round commitments to lose weight and prevent future weight gain."

Dr. Murray's warning is supported by a second report, also based on a study published in the *New England Journal of Medicine* that determined that 13 types of cancer were linked to excess body weight. Commenting on that study, Dr. Richard Wender, chief cancer control officer at the American Cancer Society (ACS), has stated that obesity and physical inactivity could someday account for more cancer deaths than smoking if the current trend toward greater rates of obesity continues.

In addition to many forms of cancer, it's long been known that obesity is directly linked to other leading causes of death in the U.S., including heart disease, stroke, hypertension, and type 2 diabetes, and that the risk of developing such conditions significantly increases due to obesity. Research also shows that obesity is a major cause of sleep apnea, osteoarthritis, depression, kidney problems, and various common gastrointestinal and respiratory conditions, along with erectile dysfunction in men. Being overweight or obese also significantly increases the risk of dying prematurely.

Clearly, then, if you are overweight, losing weight and maintaining healthy weight loss is essential for improving your health and lowering your risk of developing such conditions. In this chapter you will learn how adding coconuts and coconut oil to your diet can help you do so.

WHY LOSING WEIGHT CAN BE SO DIFFICULT

Before we explore how and why coconuts and coconut oil can aid in weight loss, let's first examine why people become overweight or obese in the first place, and why they have trouble slimming down.

The simple, commonly accepted answer is that unhealthy weight gain occurs as a result of taking in more calories each day than our bodies utilize, or burn up, to produce energy. According to this viewpoint, if you eat too much and don't burn enough calories through exercise and other types of physical activity, you will get and stay fat. That's true, as far as it goes, but it's not the entire story. Let me explain.

Calories are defined as units of heat that are used to indicate the amount of energy that foods will produce in the human body. Put simply, the foods and beverages we consume are converted by our bodies into energy. How much energy foods and beverages produce are measured in calories.

Body's Energy Needs

Your body's energy needs vary according to various factors. Such factors as the amount and intensity of the physical activity you engage in each day, whether you are sleeping or awake, your age (young people on average have a greater need for energy than older people), the type of occupation one has (physical laborers, for example, have a greater need for energy than do people who work sedentary desk jobs), and whether you are male or female.

Calories

As you eat and drink your body meets its energy needs from the calories in the foods and beverages you consume. As those energy needs are met, any remaining calories that are not converted into energy are stored in your body as fat. Specifically, this storage of calories occurs in fat cells. When this caloric storage is ongoing due to the excess consumption of food and beverages beyond your body's need for energy it leads to weight gain as well as fat-related conditions, such as a "pot belly," "love handles," and cellulite.

Taking into consideration the factors that play a role in our bodies' daily energy needs, researchers have determined that, on average, men require between 2,200 to 3,200 calories each day, while women require between 2,000 to 2,800 calories per day. These figures can increase or decrease, of course, depending on one's height, age, and daily level of physical activity.

Researchers have also determined that every pound of fat stored in our bodies is approximately equal to 3,500 calories. That same amount of calories must be "burned up" in order to lose that one pound of weight. This fact is what makes losing weight so difficult to achieve for most people who need to do so. To understand why, we need to consider another factor regarding calories. It is known as the *basal metabolic rate,* or BMR.

Basal Metabolic Rate (BMR)

The BMR is used as a measure for determining the rate at which the human body needs to burn calories in order to meet its energy demands when it is not engaged in any type of physical activity, such as when you are lying down and awake but otherwise not doing anything besides breathing. In this state, your body is performing only the basic metabolic functions required to keep it alive, and nothing more. In order to have enough energy to meet any additional level of physical activity, however, your body requires additional calories to burn.

Researchers estimate that approximately two-thirds of the calories our bodies burn each day are used to maintain our BMR. Individual BMR varies in much the same way that a person's daily caloric needs do, and for many of the same reasons, or factors, mentioned above. Now that you know what BMR is, let's return to why losing weight can be difficult.

Losing Weight

To lose a pound of weight you need to either burn approximately 3500 calories, or else eliminate that same amount of calories from your diet. The easiest way to do so might be by reducing your daily caloric intake by 500 calories. Doing so for seven consecutive days would result in the loss of one pound of weight. If you reduced your daily caloric intake by 1,000 calories, you would lose two pounds after one week. This sounds simple enough but achieving this goal for many people presents a major challenge, one that is directly due to BMR.

Remember, two-thirds of your daily caloric intake is burned as fuel in order to meet your body's basic metabolic functions. For the average adult male that means that between slightly less than 1475 to slightly more than 2100 calories must be used for this purpose. For women, on average the calories needed to be burned for this purpose are between approximately 1340 and 1875 calories. That means that even reducing 500 calories each day leaves you with fewer calories to burn in order to meet your energy needs above your basic metabolic rate. And reducing 1,000 calories from your diet each day for most people for any length of time is even more challenging and problematic. Attempting to do so can soon make them feel as if they are starving and cause them to give up trying to lose weight.

Further compounding the problem of weight loss is the difference between simply losing weight and losing weight in the form of body fat. They aren't necessarily the same thing. The rapid weight loss touted by so many quick-fix diets and weight loss products, for example, most often results in a loss of water, not fat, in the body.

In some cases, these approaches can also result in a loss of muscle mass, which is not at all healthy. Nor is losing water weight necessarily. As doing so can result in a state of chronic, low-grade dehydration, which has been linked to a wide range of health problems, including, ironically, unhealthy weight gain.

The goal for healthy weight loss is to lose body fat while retaining and, if necessary, adding muscle mass. Doing so results in a healthy body mass index (BMI). It makes it easier to keep excess weight off, unlike most diets and weight loss products, which all too often result in people regaining all of the weight they lost, and even more, after people stop dieting and using such products. This is why most physicians and weight loss experts advise a slowly-but-surely approach to losing weight. Such an approach not only makes it easier to achieve your weight loss goals, it will also result in a loss of body fat and a shift in your BMI so that you also reduce your risk of developing the wide range of diseases that a high BMI score is associated with.

Perhaps the best news about such an approach is that it does not rely on counting calories. Instead, it emphasizes making small, yet effective changes in the types of foods you eat, along with a moderate increase in the amount of exercise or other physical activities you engage in each day. As the rest of this chapter will show you, adding coconuts and coconut oil to your daily diet can improve the effectiveness of this type of weight loss plan and enhance its benefits even further.

Macronutrients and the Number of Calories They Supply

The foods you eat are made up of one or more classes of macronutrients—proteins, carbohydrates, and fats. It is from these macronutrients that your body obtains the calories it requires to meet its energy needs.

Researchers have determined that every gram of protein provides approximately four calories. The same amount of calories is provided in every gram of carbohydrate. By contrast, a gram of fat supplies more than double the amount of calories, approximately nine calories. This is why many diet plans call for people who need to lose weight to reduce the amount of fat they consume each day; doing so for any extended period of time, however, can be difficult for most people. Moreover, it can also be unhealthy, depending on the types of fats that are reduced or eliminated from one's diet. That's because, as you learned in Chapter 2, fats are essential for good health, just as proteins and carbohydrates are.

When it comes to fats and weight loss, the key is not to reduce your fat intake so much as it is to choose the types of fats you consume wisely, so that you obtain the healthy fats your body needs, such as those found in coconuts and coconut oil. Try avoiding unhealthy trans-fats and an excess of omega-6 fatty acids.

HOW COCONUTS AND COCONUT OIL
CAN HELP YOU LOSE WEIGHT AND KEEP IT OFF

Weight loss experts have long known that there are three interrelated factors that are necessary in order for people to successfully lose weight and keep it off: appetite control, improved or increased metabolism, and the conversion of energy derived from food into heat, a process known as diet-induced thermogenesis.

Appetite Control

Appetite control is self-explanatory. It means not overeating so that you do not consume an excessive amount of calories from your daily meals. Excess caloric intake leads to excess weight. Controlling one's appetite can be difficult for some people, however. Often the failure to control appetite is explained by a lack of willpower, but this isn't truly the case. Many instances of overeating occur simply because a person still feels hungry due to the body producing hunger pangs. Ironically, hunger pangs can be quite common among people who are overweight even after overeating.

Metabolism

People who struggle to lose weight also tend to have a sluggish metabolism. Metabolism refers to how your body breaks down the foods and drinks you consume into their component parts (primarily proteins in the form of amino acids, carbohydrates, and fats) so that your body can then use them to sustain itself and produce energy. People who have a normal, efficient metabolism typically do not have a problem maintaining their weight at a healthy level, while people with a low, or sluggish, metabolism struggle to avoid unhealthy weight gain.

Thermogenesis

Thermogenesis is the term used to describe the conversion of energy into heat. Diet-induced thermogenesis refers to the energy required to digest and assimilate the foods we eat that is measured as an increase in body heat production as foods are metabolized. During the metabolic process a portion of dietary calories in excess of those needed to meet your body's immediate energy requirements are converted into heat instead of being stored as fat. On average, diet-induced thermogeneis equals about ten percent of our bodies' total daily energy expenditure and is related to the type and amount of food we consume.

Thermogenesis is a crucial factor in regulating your body weight, along with your basal metabolic rate and your daily level of physical activity. It accounts for all the energy your body expends when you are resting above and beyond your BMR. High diet-induced thermogenesis helps maintain healthy weight and aids in promoting weight loss. People who are overweight or obese often have a defect in this process of thermogenesis and are therefore more prone to gain weight and have problems shedding excess pounds.

BENEFIT OF ADDING COCONUTS AND COCONUT OIL TO YOUR DIET

The inclusion of coconuts and, especially, coconut oil in your diet can go a long way toward addressing each of the above three factors and improve your ability to maintain a healthy weight and, if necessary, lose unwanted pounds. Once again, the medium-chain fatty acids (MCFAs) that coconut and its oil contain are the key.

Coconut's MCFAs Help Appetite Control

Unlike long-chain fatty acids (LCFAs), research has shown that when MCFAs are added to the diet, they create greater feelings of satiety (feeling full), which in turn leads a reduction in food consumption and therefore calories, all without any need for willpower. This has been confirmed by a number of research studies.

One such study dates back to 1996 and was published in the *International Journal of Obesity*. The study was conducted over three phases, each lasting for 14 days. In all three phases a group of men were provided high fat meals and allowed to eat as much as they wanted each day. In the first 14 days, 20 percent of the fats in each meal consisted of MCFAs and 40 percent of the fats were LCFAs. In the second phase meals consisted of equal amounts of MCFAs and LCFAs, and in the third phase MCFAs provided 40 percent of the fats in the meals the men ate, with an additional 20 percent of fats provided by LCFAs. The researchers found that the amount of food and therefore the amount of calories that the men consumed each day continued to be reduced as the amount of MCFAs in their meals was increased. The greatest reduction in food and calorie consumption occurred during the third phase in which the amount of MCFAs in their meals was highest.

Follow-up human studies have produced similar results confirming MCFAs' ability to satisfy hunger and reduce food and calorie consumption. The results of two of the more significant of these studies were published in the *European Journal of Clinical Nutrition* in 2014. In both studies, overweight men were randomly divided into two groups. At breakfast, the men received either 20 grams of MCFAs or 20 grams of LCFAs. In the first study, the men then ate lunch three hours later, while in the second test the men were given an additional 10 grams of either MCFAs or LCFAs one hour before lunch. In both tests the men's blood was also tested over a three hour period. In both studies researchers found that consumption of MCFAs "reduced food intake [and thus calorie consumption] acutely." Moreover, the studies also found that MCFAs also reduced the rise of glucose (sugar) and triglycerides after the men ate. This is important because both glucose and triglycerides levels typically rise after meals, triggering inflammation in the body.

Coconut MCFAs Boost Metabolism and Improve Diet-Induced Thermogenesis

Metabolism and diet-induced thermogenesis are closely related. Your body's metabolic rate is determined by measuring how much energy it expends to burn calories. This is known as energy expenditure, or EE. In a well-functioning metabolism, EE is higher and more calories are burned at a higher rate, leaving fewer calories to be stored as fat. When this happens it means that there is a greater thermogenic effect, as well.

Studies dating back to the 1980s and 1990s have documented that MCFAs, such as those found in coconuts and coconut oil, can significantly increase EE and therefore boost metabolism and improve thermogenesis when taken with or before meals. This, in turn, results in more calories being burned up to produce energy rather than being converted into fat.

A study published in 1986 was among the first to demonstrate the beneficial effects of MCFAs taken with meals in contrast to long-chain fatty acids (LCFAs). In this study the metabolic and thermogenic effects of MCFAs and LCFAs were compared when either MCFAs or LCFAs were added to meals consumed by seven healthy males. The participants' metabolic rate was measured both before the meals were consumed and then six hours after they ate their meals. Also measured before and after meals was the men's mean rate of oxygen consumption. (Oxygen consumption typically increases after we eat. The rate by which it increases is a sign of how well a person's metabolism is working. Higher rates of oxygen consumption after meals correspond to a healthier metabolism.) Following their meals, the men's rate of thermogenesis was also evaluated using a process known as indirect calorimetry, a method for measuring changes in heat that is produced as food is metabolized. The study found that consuming MCFAs with meals increased the participant's rate of oxygen consumption by 12 percent, compared to only a 4 percent increase when LCFAs were included with meals.

In addition, when MCFA's were included in meals the study's researchers reported that there was "a 25-fold increase in plasma beta-hydroxybutyrate concentration." Beta-hydroxybutyrate is a type of ketone. Ketones, as you learned in Chapter 5, are substances that supply energy to the body without the need for insulin to process glucose into energy. This significant increase in beta-hydroxybutyrate indicates that the inclusion of MCFAs produces a ketogenic effect. In recent years, an increasing number of health experts have begun recommending a ketogenic diet for weight loss and as a tool for reducing the risk of cancer, diabetes, and other conditions. There was no increase of beta-hydroxybutyrate following meals with LCFAs, demonstrating that LCFAs have no ketogenic benefits.

Another important finding of this study was that when LCFAs were added to meals, they caused a spike in triglycerides levels by an average of 68 percent. Not only is an increase in triglycerides an indication of inflammation in the body, it is also a serious risk factor for heart disease. By contrast, there was no change in the men's triglycerides levels when they ate meals with MCFAs.

In another study, published in 1991, a group of six obese men and six men with a lean body weight were given either 38 grams of LCFAs or 30 grams of MCFAs combined with 8 grams of LCFAs mixed into their meals. Prior to eating the metabolic rate of both groups of men was assessed. Following their meals their metabolic rate as well as their level of diet-induced thermogenesis were then measured in six-hour intervals. The researchers found that in both groups of men those who were given the combination of MCFAs and LCFAs had a higher resting metabolic rate base and increased levels of diet-induced thermogenesis based on an assessment of their energy expenditure. In the lean body weight group the men's EE increased by an average of 48 percent, while there was an even higher increase in the EE of the men who were obese. In that group EE increased by an average of 65 percent, demonstrating that the metabolic and thermogenic effects of MCFAs for people who are overweight are even greater than they are for people who are not overweight. No such benefits were achieved by either group of men who were given LCFAs with their meals.

Subsequent research has demonstrated that the metabolic and thermogenic benefits of MCFAs are long-lasting. This is true when even low amounts of MCFAs are taken before or with meals. Researchers have shown that simply adding low to moderate amounts of MCFAs to a single meal each day can boost overall metabolism for 24 hours. In addition, researchers have also discovered that if people who are overweight made it a point of replacing all LCFA-rich oils in their diet with MCFA oils, of which coconut oil has the highest concentrations, this one single step alone could result in as much as 36 pounds of weight lost within one year without dieting.

Since coconuts and coconut oil are the richest food sources of MCFAs, based on these studies you can understand why making coconuts and coconut oil a part of your daily diet can pay big dividends when it comes to achieving and maintaining a healthy weight.

Coconut Oil Can Help Reduce Belly Fat

One of the most dangerous risk factors for the diseases associated with being overweight or obese is the accumulation of fat around the abdomen and the organs of the body located in this region. There are two types of "belly fat." The first type is known as *subcutaneous* belly fat, which refers to fat stored just beneath the surface of the skin. This is the type of belly fat that you can pinch with your fingers. In most people, subcutaneous belly fat ends up being deposited in the hips and thighs rather than the abdomen.

The second type is known as *visceral* or "deep" belly fat, which refers to fat stored further beneath the skin and which wraps itself around organs, such as the kidneys, liver, and pancreas. Nearly all fat associated with excess weight in the abdominal area consists of visceral fat. Visceral belly fat triggers both insulin resistance and chronic inflammation in the body and has been linked to a greater risk for a wide variety of disease conditions, including arthritis, cancer, dementia, diabetes, heart disease, stroke, sleeping disorders, and sexual dysfunction. Excess weight gain around the abdomen, such as a "beer belly" and/or "love handles," is a sure sign of visceral belly fat. For some people who are overweight visceral belly fat is also often the most difficult type of fat to lose, persisting in the abdomen and its surrounding organs even when fat reduction in other areas of the body is achieved. Research has shown that taking coconut oil can help reduce belly fat and also shrink weight size.

One such study involved 40 overweight women between the ages of 20 and 40. The women were randomly assigned into one of two groups. Both groups followed the same type of low-calorie diet throughout the course of the study, which lasted for 12 weeks, and they also walked for 50 minutes each day. The first group of women also consumed 30 mL (approximately two tablespoons) of soybean oil each day, while the second group daily consumed 30 mL of coconut oil. All of the women in both groups were tested one week prior to the study beginning and the collected data from the testing showed no differences in the biochemical characteristics and body fat compositions between each group of women. Both groups of women were then evaluated one week after the conclusion of the 12-week period.

The results of the study found that both groups of women achieved a reduction in their body mass index (BMI). However, only the women who consumed the coconut oil achieved a reduction in their waist size. Moreover, the women who consumed soybean oil also exhibited an increase in their total LDL ("bad") cholesterol levels, and a decrease in their HDL ("good") cholesterol levels, resulting in an increase in their LDL/HDL cholesterol ratios. By contrast, the women who consumed coconut oil daily exhibited no negative changes in their total, LDL, and HDL cholesterol levels, nor a negative change in their LDL/HDL ratios. Based on these findings, the authors of the study wrote, "It appears that dietetic supplementation with coconut oil does not cause dyslipidemia [unhealthy changes in cholesterol levels] and seems to promote a reduction in abdominal obesity."

A similar study involving men also confirmed the ability of coconut oil to reduce belly fat. In this study, which involved 20 obese but otherwise healthy men between the ages of 20 and 60. Thirty mL of virgin coconut oil (VCO) was consumed by all of the men for a period of four weeks. One week prior to the study, the men's weight, body mass index, lipid profiles, and overall health of their organs were measured. The men also provided information on their total food consumption in the 24-hour period before this assessment, as well as the level of physical activity that they had engaged in the four weeks prior to the assessment. They were then instructed to continue to engage in the same amount of physical activity for the duration of the study, and to continue to eat as they had done the day before the assessment. They were also instructed to drink an adequate amount of water each day throughout the study period. The only change to their overall diet and lifestyle was the daily addition of coconut oil.

One week after the four-week period all of the participants were then tested as before. The researchers found that simply by adding the coconut oil to their daily dietary and physical activity routines the men lost an average of 2.86 centimeters (approximately 1.1 inches) from around their waist, with no negative changes to their lipid profiles. In concluding their study, the researchers wrote, "VCO is a cheap oil source containing high concentration of MCFAs which in the current study had shown beneficial effect in WC [waist circumference] reduction especially in males without any deleterious [harmful] effect to the lipid profile. VCO is also safe to use for the period of study without any deleterious effects on biochemical and organ functions."

The results of these and similar studies clearly show that the daily addition of coconut oil to your diet can help to improve your ability to lose belly fat, and therefore decrease your risk of developing the various diseases that are associated with excess belly fat.

Another Important Weight-Loss Benefit of Coconut's MCFAs

One of the main reasons why a low fat-diet is often recommended for people who need to lose weight is because fats, in comparison to proteins and carbohydrates, contain more calories. In addition, most fats, once they are consumed, are broken down into the fatty acids they contain. The fatty acids then combine with proteins to become lipoproteins (*lipo* refers to lipid, another name for fat). These lipoproteins then enter the bloodstream, depositing the fatty acids they contain into the body's fat cells. Meanwhile, the proteins and carbohydrates from the foods we eat are also broken down so that the calories they contain can be converted into energy and put to immediate use sustaining the body and its many functions. Only when carbohydrates and proteins are eaten in excess are the surplus of calories they contain converted into fat instead of energy. Otherwise, protein and carbohydrate calories supply our bodies with energy, while calories from fats are stored as fat, with one important exception.

Unlike other fats, MCFAs do not pair with proteins to become lipoproteins, nor do they circulate in the bloodstream to wind up being stored in the body's fat cells. Instead, as soon as they are consumed, MCFAs pass through to the liver, which goes to work to convert them into immediate, readily available forms of energy. This means that you do not have to be concerned about how much MCFAs you consume, unlike other types of fats, because MCFAs do not lead to fat buildup in the body. Instead, they are quickly burned to supply your body with energy, which is one more reason why MCFAs have been shown to successfully boost metabolism and thermogenesis. Moreover, MCFAs contain slightly less calories (approximately three percent) than other types of fats.

In addition, by increasing the amount of MCFAs you consume—something you can easily do by adding coconuts and coconut oil to your meals—you can spare yourself of the pitfalls of following a low-fat diet. Though for overweight people such a diet was long the standard recommended diet. Today an increasing number of physicians and weight loss specialists caution against it, and with good reason. First, as you learned in Chapter 2, fats are essential nutrients for good health. Without enough fats in our diets, we would quickly begin to develop certain nutritional deficiencies. It is through fats in foods that our bodies are supplied with vital, fat-soluble nutrients, such as carotenes and vitamins A, D, E, and K.

In addition, low-fat diets are difficult to stick to for any length of time. As human beings, we are designed to enjoy a certain amount of fat in our meals each day. Depriving ourselves of fat is not only not enjoyable, it can also leave us feeling tired and experiencing persistent hunger pangs. In a very real sense, low-fat diets can mimic the feelings of starvation. That's why most people, if they are able to achieve their weight loss goals by following a low-fat diet, proceed to regain their lost weight, and often even more, once they stop dieting.

The bottom line is that limiting your fat intake if you need to lose weight is unwise. The better solution is not to limit fats, but to choose the right fats that will support your weight loss goals and provide you with the energy you need. As this chapter makes clear, the right fats are MCFAs, and the best way to obtain them is by eating coconuts and using coconut oil for cooking and baking.

CONCLUSION

Now that you have read this chapter, if you or your loved ones need to manage your weight I hope you will consider adding coconuts to the foods you eat, and to start using coconut oil for your baking and cooking needs. You can also gain coconut oil's weight loss benefits by consuming one or two tablespoons of it each day, either all at once before breakfast, or in divided doses before breakfast, lunch, and dinner. Doing so will help you feel full and satisfied, making it easier to not overeat.

In addition to adding coconut and its oil to your weight loss regimen, be sure to get enough exercise each day. You do not have to engage in strenuous exercise or even go to the gym. Research has shown that, for most people, simply taking a 20 to 30 minute walk each day can lead to gradual, sustained weight loss over time. Also be sure to drink plenty of pure, filtered water each day to avoid developing chronic, low-grade dehydration, which is another underlying factor that can lead to unhealthy weight gain.

Now let's turn our attention in Chapter 9, to another area of concern for so many men, women, and children today—the health of their gums and teeth. That is the topic of Chapter 9.

9.

Healthy Gums and Teeth

Here is an important yet often overlooked fact that you need to know: The health of your teeth and gums has a direct bearing on your overall health. In this chapter, you will learn how coconuts, and especially coconut oil, can improve the appearance of your teeth while also preventing and reversing bacterial gum infections. First, let's look at why your dental health is so important.

THE LINK BETWEEN YOUR TEETH, GUMS, AND OVERALL HEALTH

The relationship between your teeth and the health of all of your body's systems is something that has been recognized and taught for centuries by practitioners of acupuncture and traditional Chinese medicine (TCM). As you may know, TCM teaches that energy pathways, known as meridians, travel along the length of the body, with each meridian corresponding to a specific organ system. Research by scientists in both the U.S. and Europe began to confirm the existence of the meridian pathways starting in the mid- to late 20th century.

According to TCM theory, when the flow of vital energy, known as *Qi* (pronounced "chee"), becomes imbalanced as it travels along the meridians the end result is disease. One of the factors that can cause the flow of this vital energy to become disrupted according to the TCM system of healing is the health of the teeth. For example, TCM teaches that molars that are misaligned or have cavities can interfere with the health of meridians of the stomach or intestine systems and the organs associated with them. These meridians govern not only the stomach and intestines, but also the bladder, breasts, kidneys and spleen (the stomach meridian), and the heart, lung, liver, and gallbladder (small and large intestine meridians).

Research by Western scientists appears to support these TCM teachings. In fact, some scientists now estimate that as much as half of all of the chronic and degenerative diseases plaguing today's modern world are either directly or indirectly caused by dental problems, such as cavities, infections, and tooth misalignments, as well as some of the dental procedures used to treat such problems, especially dental amalgam fillings that contain mercury and other materials may be at the source. In addition, in recent years, a growing body of scientific research has shown that plaque buildup on the teeth and bacterial infections on and beneath the gums can increase the risk of heart disease and also increase the burden on the body's immune system. For these reasons, as well as in the interests of basic hygiene, proper dental care needs to be an ongoing part of your overall health regimen.

Gum Disease and Cancer

In addition to the link researchers have established between gum disease and an increased risk of developing heart disease, scientists have now discovered that gum disease, once thought of as a fairly benign condition, can also increase your risk of certain types of cancer. In a study published in the medical journal *Lancet Oncology,* researchers tracked male health professionals for nearly two decades. All of the health professionals had a history of gum disease. By the end of the study, researchers found that the health professionals had, on average, a 14 percent overall greater risk of developing cancer compared to men who do not have gum disease.

According to lead researcher Dr. Dominique Michaud, "After controlling for smoking and other risk factors, periodontal disease was significantly associated with an increased risk of lung, kidney, pancreatic, and hematological [blood] cancers." In addition, periodontal disease was a higher than normal risk factor, even among health professionals in the study who never smoked. (Smoking can cause gum disease and is, of course, another significant risk factor for cancer.)

Prior to this study, researchers had established that people with gum disease also show a higher level of inflammation in their blood. Inflammation is now well-known to be a risk factor for certain types of cancer (as well as heart disease, diabetes, and many other health conditions). But until the *Lancet Oncology* study many researchers speculated that whatever causes inflammation in the body might also cause gum disease and cancer independently of each other.

The aim of the study conducted by Dr. Michaud and his colleagues was to determine whether or not gum disease by itself increases the risk of cancer. In order to conduct their study they used data from a previous large study of male doctors and other health professionals aged 40 to 75. That study began in 1986 at Harvard University. In it, nearly 50,000 men filled out health surveys and were followed for more than 17 years. The surveys included information on gum disease and bone loss, as well as various other criteria, such as their number of teeth and tooth loss.

Over 5,700 of the health professionals developed cancer during the time that they were tracked, not including cases of non-melanoma skin cancers and non-aggressive prostate cancer. In addition to finding that men who had gum disease had a 14 percent higher cancer risk compared to those who did not, Dr. Michaud and his team found that their risks were higher depending on the type of cancer. Among the findings of Dr. Michaud and his team were that men with a history of gum disease had a 36 percent greater risk of lung cancer, a 49 percent higher risk of kidney cancer, a 54 percent higher risk of pancreatic cancer, and a 30 percent higher risk of blood cancers (such as non-Hodgkin lymphoma, leukemia or multiple myeloma) compared to men who did not have gum disease. In addition, men who had who had fewer than the normal number of teeth (0 to 16) at the start of the study had a 70 percent higher risk of lung cancer compared with individuals with more normal teeth numbers (25 to 32).

The findings of Dr. Michaud and his team build upon previous research dating back to 1990 that showed gum disease and tooth loss can increase the risk of oral cancers. Subsequent research that followed that of Dr. Michaud also indicates that poor dental health can increase cancer risk. Such research also appears to validate the findings of the late Josef M. Issels, MD (November 21, 1907 to February 11, 1998), a pioneering integrative cancer doctor who decades ago stated that "97 percent of all cancers have a causal relationship to the mouth, teeth, jaw, and tonsil."

Gum Disease

For most people, gum disease is the biggest dental factor affecting their overall health. Also known as periodontal disease, gum disease is characterized by inflammation or degeneration of the tissues that surround and support the teeth—gingiva (gums), the bone the teeth are set in (alveolar bone), the periodontal ligament, and the cementum (the tissue that connects these structures). It is estimated that nearly 50 percent of the U.S. population suffers from some degree of gum disease. Gum disease is primarily due to poor dental hygiene (lack of teeth brushing and flossing) and poor diet, leading to a buildup of bacterial plaque.

The most common and often initial form of gum disease is inflammation of the gums, called gingivitis. If left untreated, gingivitis can spread, causing increased inflammation in the membranes and tissues around the base of the teeth and potential erosion of the underlying bone, a condition known as periodontitis. Periodontitis is the major cause of bone and tooth loss in adults. The most common symptom of gum disease is red, inflamed gum tissue that bleeds easily due to flossing, brushing of the teeth, and/or eating hard foods such as raw apples.

The bacteria associated with plaque buildup and gum disease can migrate to other parts of the body by entering the bloodstream via the capillaries in

Gum Disease
Linked to Alzheimer's Disease

Recent research has now established a link between Alzheimer's disease and dementia, as well as other impairments of cognitive (mental) function. This link has been outlined in a number of studies, including a study conducted by researchers at the University of Southampton and King's College London, England. Their findings were published in 2016 in *PLOS ONE,* a peer-reviewed medical journal published by the Public Library of Science.

In the introduction to their study the researchers wrote, "Periodontitis is common in the elderly and may become more common in Alzheimer's disease because of a reduced ability to take care of oral hygiene as the disease progresses. Elevated antibodies to periodontal bacteria are associated with an increased systemic pro-inflammatory state. Elsewhere, raised serum pro-inflammatory cytokines have been associated with an increased rate of cognitive decline in Alzheimer's disease." Knowing this, the researchers set out to determine "if periodontitis in Alzheimer's disease is associated with both increased dementia severity and cognitive decline, and an increased systemic pro-inflammatory state."

The study involved 59 participants suffering with mild to moderate Alzheimer's disease. The cognitive function of all of the participants was assessed at the beginning of the study and a blood sample from each participant was taken to measure their bodies' inflammation levels. The participants' dental health was also assessed by a dental hygienist who gum tissue. As bacteria that originate in the mouth spreads elsewhere in the body, it can cause or worsen a variety of illnesses. In addition to heart disease, a number of other chronic, degenerative conditions, including diabetes, pulmonary (lung) disease, gastrointestinal problems, and low-birth-weight complications in pregnancy have been linked to periodontal disease by scientific research. Researchers have also established a link between periodontal disease and certain type of cancer (see Gum Disease and Cancer on page 138).

Additional research has also established a link between gum disease and rheumatoid arthritis. Gum disease has also been linked to Alzheimer's disease and dementia (*see* Gum Disease Linked To Alzheimer's Disease on page 140). Chronic inflammation caused by the bacterial infections that cause gum disease is the primary reason poor oral health can lead to such serious diseases.

---

was not told of the participants' levels of cognitive function. Six months later all of these assessments were repeated.

The study found that gum disease was associated with a 600 percent increase in the rate of cognitive decline in the participants over the six-month period of the study, and that periodontitis was also linked with an increase in the participants' overall levels of inflammation over the same period. As a result of their findings, the researchers concluded that gum disease is indeed linked to an increase in cognitive decline in patients with Alzheimer's disease, and that this increase is likely due to the body's inflammatory response to oral bacteria and other harmful microorganisms.

Commenting on the study, one of its authors, Dr. Mark Ide, stated, "A number of studies have shown that having few teeth, possibly as a consequence of earlier gum disease, is associated with a greater risk of developing dementia. Based on various research findings, we also believe that the presence of teeth with active gum disease results in higher body-wide levels of the sorts of inflammatory molecules which have also been associated with an elevated risk of other outcomes, such as cognitive decline or cardiovascular disease. Research has suggested that effective gum treatment can reduce the levels of these molecules closer to that seen in a healthy state.

"Previous studies have also shown that patients with Alzheimer's disease have poorer dental health than others of similar age and that the more severe the dementia the worse the dental health, most likely reflecting greater difficulties with taking care of oneself as dementia becomes more severe."

The best treatment for gum disease is prevention, which includes brushing your teeth and flossing after each meal, and seeing a holistic dentist for checkups every six months. Coconut oil can also help maintain the health of your teeth and gums, including helping to reverse gum disease and plaque buildup.

COCONUT OIL AS A DENTAL AID

Adding coconut oil to your daily dental care regimen can help improve the appearance of your teeth and help prevent and reverse the buildup of harmful bacteria on both your teeth and gums. The use of coconut oil as a dental aid has been recommended for many centuries by practitioners of Ayurvedic medicine, also known as Ayurveda, which developed in India thousands of years ago. Ayurveda is recognized by the World Health Organization (WHO) as a viable system of medicine. WHO also supports ongoing research into Ayurveda and recommends it be a part of comprehensive modern medical approach to health.

Like traditional Chinese medicine, Ayurveda has long recognized the important links between dental and overall health. One of its oldest texts, known as the *Charaka Sambita*, which was written approximately three thousand years ago, first made mention of coconut oil as an aid to dental health. Ayurveda teaches that the use of coconut oil can help keep teeth white and healthy and prevent and help eliminate harmful microorganisms in the mouth that contribute to plaque buildup and gum infections. Today, research is verifying what Ayurvedic physicians have known for centuries.

As you learned in chapters 2 and 6, many of the nutrients that coconuts and coconut oil contain are known to protect against harmful microorganisms. Research shows that this includes unhealthy bacteria responsible for plaque buildup and gum disease and infection. As you also learned, the principal ingredients in coconuts and coconut oil that are most responsible for protecting against harmful bacteria and other microorganisms are the medium chain fatty acids (MCFAs) they contain, especially lauric acid, which makes up approximately 50 percent of the MCFAs found in coconut.

MCFAs Fight Harmful Mouth Bacteria

Research has demonstrated that lauric acid and coconut's other MCFAs have proven antibacterial, as well as anti-inflammatory properties. Moreover, these MCFAs tend to seek out and eliminate harmful bacteria while leaving beneficial bacteria intact. This is important when it comes to your dental health because your mouth, like the rest of your body, plays host to a variety of bacteria and other microorganisms, some of which play vital roles in maintaining the health of your gums and teeth, and some of which do just the opposite. For example, one of the most beneficial bacteria found in the mouth is *Streptococcus salivarius*. It not only helps to maintain the health of gums and teeth, it also helps prevent halitosis (bad breath) and plays a vital role in maintaining the health of the upper respiratory tract.

By contrast, another member of the strep family of bacteria, *Streptococcus mutans*, acts as a primary cause of tooth decay and cavities, as well as gum disease. The presence of *Streptococcus mutans* in the mouth is quite common today, since it is aided in its spread in the mouth by the consumption of sugars and starchy foods, as well as poor dental hygiene. As it spreads, it not only harms teeth and gums, it can migrate deeper into the body to cause harm to the heart and its arteries, as well as to the brain.

Two other harmful bacteria that are typically found in cases of poor oral health are *P. Gingivalis* and *A. Acitomycetemcomitans*, both of which have been shown by scientific research to cause rheumatoid arthritis once they pass from the mouth to enter the body's bloodstream. These bacteria typically take root in connective tissue near bone, including the jawbone. Once they gain a foothold in the mouth or body they release an enzyme that alters certain body proteins. Over time, as these proteins continue to be altered, they progressively damage the connective tissue near bone and the body's immune system no longer recognizes them as belonging to the body. Instead, the immune system targets and attacks them as harmful invaders. As the immune system's attack progresses it can impact the health and stability of connective tissues, causing bone damage in the jawbone, and potentially tooth loss and damage to joints in the body that is a hallmark of rheumatoid arthritis.

Due to its overall antimicrobial properties coconut oil can help prevent and reverse the colonization of such harmful bacteria in your gums, teeth, and mouth. There are two ways you can obtain the benefits of coconut oil for this purpose. You can use it as toothpaste or as an alternative to commercial mouthwash products using an Ayurvedic technique known as "oil pulling."

Coconut Oil Toothpaste

You can easily make your own toothpaste using coconut oil. For best results, choose organic, extra virgin coconut oil for this purpose. Like all other saturated fats, coconut oil is solid at room temperature. It typically turns liquid at a temperature of 76 degrees Fahrenheit (24 degrees Centigrade) and above. If your home is below that temperature, simply scoop out a teaspoon of coconut oil and warm it up. Once it is in liquid form, place a few drops on your toothbrush, making sure that enough coconut oil coats all of the toothbrush's bristles. Then brush your teeth as you normally would. Be sure to allow the coconut oil to reach and penetrate into your gum line. When you are finished brushing, clean your toothbrush thoroughly by rinsing it in warm water and also rinse your mouth.

You can also make toothpaste using equal parts organic, extra virgin coconut oil and baking soda. Apply the coconut oil to your toothbrush first and then apply the baking soda. If you choose to try this method, be sure to use a baking soda product that does not contain aluminum.

By using coconut oil to brush your teeth you will be providing your teeth and gums with its antibacterial properties. Over time, you may also experience some degree of whitening of your teeth without the need to use commercial teeth whitening products that can contain harsh chemicals.

Once you finish brushing your teeth you can also massage your gums with coconut oil to further enhance its gum-protecting benefits.

Oil Pulling With Coconut Oil

Oil pulling has been a traditional dental remedy within the Ayurvedic system of healing for approximately 3,000 years. Known as *Kavala graha* or *Gandoosha* in India, where it is widely practiced, oil pulling was first written about in the *Charaka Sambita*. It involves swishing liquid coconut oil (sesame oil or a combination of the two oils can also be used) in the mouth in much the same way that mouthwash products are swished to clean and protect gums from bacteria and plaque buildup. Typically, swishing is done for between 10 to 20 minutes once or twice a day, until the coconut oil becomes thin, milky white in consistency, after which it is spit out. According to the *Charaka Sambita*, the daily practice of oil pulling can not only protect the mouth, gums, and teeth from harmful bacteria and other microorganisms, it can also help eliminate toxins from elsewhere in the body.

Oil pulling with coconut oil is said to work because of how the MCFAs that coconut oil contains break down and bind with plaque-causing bacteria. The swishing process pulls the bacteria away from the gums and teeth, and the bacteria is then eliminated when the coconut oil is spit out. This process is further enhanced by the digestive enzymes contained in saliva. As saliva interacts with the coconut oil during the oil pulling process it metabolizes and activates the MCFAs that the oil contains so that they can more easily seek out, bind with, and destroy unhealthy bacteria in the mouth. This helps explains why oil pulling with coconut oil has been shown to be more effective for reducing harmful bacteria and preventing and relieving gum disease than simply using coconut oil to brush one's teeth. It also perhaps explains why oil pulling is recommended in the *Charaka Sambita* and other Ayurvedic texts as a method of oral hygiene, while using coconut oil as a tooth paste is not a common Ayurvedic process.

Now that you've read about oil pulling with coconut oil, the question you may be asking yourself is, does it really work?

Until recently, aside from anecdotal reports that it did, there was little scientific research that existed to answer that question. Now, however, scientists have started to investigate oil pulling and published studies to confirm that oil pulling does indeed help to maintain the health of gums and teeth. A number of studies, for example, have determined that oil pulling with coconut oil (as well as with sesame oil) creates a detergent-like effect known as saponification within the mouth, and that it is this effect that explains how and why oil pulling can prevent and reduce bad bacteria and plaque, maintain healthy gum tissues, and prevent bacteria in the mouth, including *Streptococcus mutans*, from entering the bloodstream to migrate deeper into the body.

In a randomized controlled study 60 test subjects were randomly divided into three groups and studied over a two-week period. Saliva samples from the participants were collected and cultured on the first day of the study and again two weeks later after the study's completion. In both saliva cultures the amount of *Streptococcus mutans* in the mouths of each participant was also assessed. During the study, the first group of participants performed oil pulling with coconut oil for ten minutes each day. The second group rinsed their mouths with chlorhexidine mouthwash (chlorhexidine is a main ingredient in many commercial mouthwash products) for one minute each day, which is the average length of time most people take when using mouthwash products. The third group acted as the control group and rinsed their mouths with distilled water for one minute each day.

At the conclusion of the study, the researchers reported that "Statistically significant reduction in *S. mutans* count was seen in both the coconut oil pulling and chlorhexidine group." leading them to conclude that "oil-pulling therapy is natural, safe and has no side effects. Hence, it can be considered as a preventive therapy at home to maintain oral hygiene."

Research has also found that oil pulling is just as effective as the use of chlorhexidine for preventing and reducing halitosis (bad breath) and eliminating the bacteria and other microorganisms that cause it.

In another study, researchers set out to explore the effectiveness of oil pulling with coconut oil as a treatment for plaque-induced gingivitis. The study involved 60 teen-aged boys and girls between the ages of 16 and 18. All of the participants were in the habit of brushing their teeth at least once a day before the study began.

The study lasted for 30 days. At the start of the study, as well as on days 7, 15, and 30, the amount of plaque and degree of gingivitis in the participants' teeth and gums were assessed using what is known as Kappa scores for modified gingival index and a plaque index. At the beginning of the study the participants' baseline mean gingival index was 0.91 and their mean plaque index was 1.19. During the study all of the participants were instructed to perform oil pulling with coconut oil every morning in addition to their normal oral hygiene routines.

The authors of the study reported that, "In comparison to the baseline values both the gingival and the plaque indices substantially reduced during the period of assessment. There was a steady decline in both the plaque index and the gingival index values from day 7. The average gingival index score on day 30 was down to 0.401 and the plaque index score was 0.385."

In other words, after only 30 days of daily oil pulling with coconut oil, there was a more than 50 percent reduction in the participants mean gingival index and a nearly two-thirds reduction in their mean plaque index, and the reduction in both index scores was apparent after only one week.

"The significant reduction in gingivitis can be attributed to decreased plaque accumulation and the anti-inflammatory, emollient effect of coconut oil," the authors of the study wrote. They concluded their study by writing, "Oil pulling has been proven to be an effective method in reducing plaque formation and plaque induced gingivitis. This preliminary study shows that coconut oil is an easily usable, safe, and cost effective agent with minimal side effects which can be used as an adjuvant in oral hygiene maintenance."

How To Perform Oil Pulling Using Coconut Oil

To start using coconut oil for oil pulling in order to cleanse your mouth, teeth, and gums be sure to select a brand of organic, extra virgin coconut oil that is free of any other additives (*see* Resources on page 177).

You can perform oil pulling once or twice a day, ideally in the morning before breakfast and again before you go to bed. Here are some guidelines to follow:

- Always perform oil pulling on an empty stomach. Wait at least four hours after you eat and between one and two hours after consuming any liquids.

- Before you begin, brush and floss your teeth and gums, scrape your tongue, and then rinse your mouth thoroughly.

- Then place two teaspoons of organic, extra virgin coconut oil in your mouth. (If it is solid, you can warm it up or simply allow it to liquefy in your mouth.)

- Hold the coconut oil in your mouth for at least ten minutes, swishing it as you would swish mouthwash. As you do so, your saliva will mix with the coconut oil to begin pulling bacteria away from your teeth, gum, and tongue. For this reason you must take care not to swallow any of the mixture while you are swishing.

- Once you are done, spit out all of the mixture. Because of the toxins that have been pulled into the mixture, it is best to spit it out into your toilet rather than your bathroom sink.

- Then rinse your mouth thoroughly with warm water.

That's all there is to it. At first, oil pulling may take some time to get used to, but as you begin to experience how clean and fresh it helps to keep your gums, teeth, and breath you will soon find that you will want to make it a regular part of your daily oral hygiene routine.

CONCLUSION

Good dental health, like your overall health in general, requires more than a single step solution. To ensure the health of your teeth and gums, be sure to see your dentist regularly (at least once a year, and more frequently if necessary). Also be sure to brush your teeth after meals, and to gently floss at least once a day. In addition, avoid sugary drinks and foods, and minimize your intake of high-starch foods, all of which create a favorable environment in your mouth for harmful bacteria and plaque to take root and grow. And now that you know of the proven health benefits coconut oil has as a dental aid, I hope you will consider trying oil pulling with coconut oil as well. At the very least, I encourage you to experiment with making a tooth paste from coconut oil with or without baking soda.

In the next chapter, you will learn how coconut oil can improve the health of your hair and skin.

10.

The Tropical Beauty Aid

Coconut oil has long been used as a beauty aid by people in the tropical regions where coconuts grow. The inhabitants there use it to maintain the health of both their hair and skin. This chapter provides tips and guidelines so that you, too, can make use of this tropical beauty aid.

HAIR CARE

Coconut oil is an excellent hair conditioner, leaving hair lustrous and shiny. In addition, coconut oil can protect hair from becoming damaged due to protein loss. In doing so, it also protects against split ends and helps keep hair from becoming too dry and/or frizzy.

Protects Hair from Protein Loss

The ability of coconut oil to protect hair from protein loss was verified in a study published in the *Journal of Cosmetic Science*. This study was a follow-up to previous studies that showed that the application of coconut oil to the hair prevented hair from becoming damaged due to combing and brushing, regardless of a person's hair type.

In the study researchers examined the hair-healing properties of coconut oil compared to both mineral oil and sunflower oil. As the researchers pointed out, mineral oil is "extensively used in hair oil formulations in India because it is non-greasy in nature, and because it is cheaper than vegetable oils like coconut and sunflower oils," whereas sunflower oil "is the second most utilized base oil in the hair oil industry." The researchers carried out a wide array of tests on the three oils in order to cover many different types of hair treatments, as well as to examine how each type of oil worked on different hair types.

Once these tests were completed and analyzed, the researchers wrote, "The findings clearly indicate the strong impact that coconut oil application has to hair as compared to application of both sunflower and mineral oils. Among the three oils, coconut oil was the only oil found to reduce the protein loss remarkably for both undamaged and damaged hair when used as a pre-wash and post-wash grooming product. Both sunflower and mineral oils do not help at all in reducing the protein loss from hair."

The benefits of coconut oil for protecting against hair protein loss was attributed to the medium chain fatty acids (MCFAs) that coconut oil contains, especially lauric acid. "Coconut oil," the researchers wrote, "being a triglyceride of lauric acid (principal fatty acid), has a high affinity for hair proteins and, because of its low molecular weight and straight linear chain, is able to penetrate inside the hair shaft. Mineral oil, being a hydrocarbon, has no affinity for proteins and therefore is not able to penetrate and yield better results. In the case of sunflower oil, although it is a triglyceride of linoleic acid, because of its bulky structure due to the presence of double bonds, it does not penetrate the fiber, consequently resulting in no favorable impact on protein loss."

Interestingly, nearly all other vegetable oils that are used by the hair care industry to manufacture shampoos and conditioners fall into the same category as sunflower oil does. All of these oils are composed of long-chain fatty acids, not MCFAs. Based on the findings of the above study, this means that coconut oil is superior to all other vegetable oils when it comes to protecting hair from damage caused by protein loss.

Prevents and Reverses Dandruff

When massaged into the scalp, coconut oil can also help prevent and reverse dandruff and other minor scalp conditions. Dandruff is caused by the shedding of dead skin cells from the scalp. The shedding of dead skin cells is a normal, natural process. However, when shedding becomes excessive, white, oily-looking flakes of dead skin can cluster in the hair and shoulders resulting in dandruff. The MCFAs coconut oil acts as a natural emollient that soothes and softens the scalp at the same time that they nourish hair, helping to prevent dandruff buildup.

Applying Coconut Oil to Your Hair and Scalp

The best and easiest way to obtain the healing benefits of coconut oil for your scalp and hair is to use one to two teaspoons of organic, extra virgin coconut oil. Apply it to your scalp and hair and then massage it thoroughly so that it coats both your hair and scalp. You can take up to five minutes or more to do this, depending on the length and thickness of your hair.

Once you finish, let the oil sit so that it completely soaks into both your scalp and hair shafts. Wait at least 20 minutes, ideally 30 minutes or more, before you gently rinse your scalp and hair with water. You may find that you prefer to do this at the start of the day. If you do so, you can also perform oil pulling with coconut oil as you let the oil soak into your hair and scalp (*see* Chapter 9).

You might find that you prefer to apply coconut oil before you go to bed, and then cover your head with a shower cap to allow the oil to soak in while you sleep. Either way, once you rinse off your hair, either over the sink or in the shower, gently damp dry your hair. By applying coconut oil to your hair and scalp one or more times each week you will soon find that doing so helps to improve the health of your scalp while strengthening and improving the look and luster of your hair.

SKIN CARE

Coconut oil has long been used as a skin cream in tropical regions where coconuts grow. In many of these regions both men and women apply coconut oil to their bodies on a daily basis, not only to keep their skin smooth and moisturized, but also to protect them against sunburn and skin infections. In recent years, the healing properties of coconut oil as a skin cream have begun to be confirmed by scientific research.

Benefits for Your Skin

There are a number of reasons why coconut oil is good for your skin.

- As mentioned above, coconut oil acts as a natural emollient to keep skin smooth and to help soothe minor abrasions and dry, patchy skin.

- Coconut oil also acts as a natural exfoliant, meaning that it helps get rid of dead skin cells. When such cells build up on the skin they can cause blemishes and leave skin looking old and dull. Once dead skin cells are removed, however, skin becomes smoother and can often regain a more youthful appearance.

- The medium-chain fatty acids in coconut oil can help reduce inflammation both internally in the body and externally, making them an effective aid for dealing with a variety of skin conditions.

- The ingredients in coconut oil help to strengthen the skin's connective tissues. By doing so, it can help prevent wrinkles and the appearance of fine lines.

- Research shows that coconut oil applied to skin can block approximately 20 percent of the sun's ultraviolet (UV) light. While this is less than the 30 percent blockage achieved by most commercial sunscreens, coconut oil is free of the toxic chemicals that such sunscreens often contain, which can be absorbed by the skin to enter the body. In addition, such sun blocking products can also interfere with how sunlight exposure produces vitamin D in the body. Vitamin D has been shown to provide a wide variety of health benefits, including protecting against many types of cancer. When coconut oil is used as a sunscreen, the body's ability to produce vitamin D from sunlight is far less impacted.

- The final word, and perhaps, most important reason is that coconut oil helps promote healthy skin is because of how similar the medium-chain fatty acids it contains are to the MCFAs found in sebum, your skin's natural oil. Sebum acts as a protective coating that covers the skin. The surface of the skin is also home to a variety of friendly bacteria. Known as *lipophilic* bacteria, these friendly bacteria are attracted to and interact with fats, including the fatty acids found in sebum.

  As these friendly bacteria interact with the MCFAs in sebum, they catalyze the MCFAs so that the MCFAs are able to resist and eliminate harmful bacteria and other microorganisms that can cause skin infections and negatively impact the appearance of skin. This same process occurs when the skin's friendly, lipophilic bacteria interact with the MCFAs contained in coconut oil, making coconut oil an effective, natural antimicrobial and antiseptic skin lotion.

Healing Properties for Your Skin

It's because of coconut oil's skin-healing properties that coconut oil is often included as an ingredient in commercial skin cream and lotion products. However, many such products also contain chemicals and other ingredients that are not necessarily healthy, making coconut oil by itself a wiser choice.

Now let's examine some of the specific benefits coconut oil provides for skin conditions.

Burns

Animal studies indicate that coconut oil can also be beneficial for treating burns, both by itself and in combination with conventional burn medications. In one such study, rats were divided into four groups, with six rats in each group. Burn wounds were inflicted on the rats in all four groups.

The first group of rats served as the control group. The second group received treatment with silver sulphadiazine, a standard burn medication. The third group was treated with virgin coconut oil, and the fourth group was treated with a combination of virgin coconut oil and silver sulphadiazine. The rats in groups two through four received once daily topical treatments for a period of 21 days or until complete healing occurred, depending on whether the healing occurred before the end of the 21-day period. The study found that there was "a significant improvement in burn wound contraction" in the group of rats who received treatments with coconut oil alone and the group that received coconut oil in combination with silver sulphadiazine. The period of time required for full re-epithelialization of the burn wound areas also decreased significantly in both of these groups. Based on these results, the study's authors wrote that coconut oil can be considered an inexpensive and effective aid added to other topical burn medications in order to "significantly enrich the assortment of topical medications available for the treatment of burns" and to attain faster healing without the risk of complications.

Cuts and Wounds

Because of its antiseptic and antibacterial properties, coconut oil can help speed the healing of cuts and wounds. Research has also found that coconut oil helps cuts and burns heal in three additional ways, as well.

1. First, it improves the activity of antioxidant enzymes that are produced by the body in response to cuts and wounds in order to protect the affected injury site from free radical damage.

2. Coconut oil has also been found to stimulate higher cross linking of collagen within the tissues affected by cuts and wounds.

3. And it also accelerates the speed in which cuts and wounds are covered with healing tissue, a process known as re-epithelialization (the new, healing tissue is known as epithelial tissue).

These three benefits coconut oil has for cuts and wounds have been confirmed by animal studies. In one such study, excision wounds were administered to three groups of rats. There were six rats in each group. The first group of rats acted as the control group. The second and third groups were administered 0.5 and 1 mL of virgin coconut oil respectively, beginning 24 hours after the wound occurred and continuing once daily for a period of 10 days. During this time the rats in all three groups were monitored to determine the amount of time it took for their wounds to close, and to determine the degree of the production and cross-linking of collagen within the wounded areas. The rats' antioxidant status during the wound healing process was also monitored continuously for 14 days.

According to the researchers, in both groups of rats to which coconut oil was applied to their wounds the wounds "healed much faster, as indicated by a decreased time of complete epithelization and higher levels of various skin components." In addition, collagen "showed a significant increase in VCO [virgin coconut oil]-treated wounds, indicating a higher collagen cross-linking." Antioxidant enzyme activities among both groups of VCO-treated rats were also found to have increased by the 10th day after wounding occurred, and then returned to normal levels by day 14. The authors of the study concluded that the beneficial healing benefits of virgin coconut oil on wounds "can be attributed to the cumulative effect of various biologically active minor components present in it [VCO]."

Dermatitis

Also known as eczema, dermatitis is a skin condition caused by inflammation of the skin's outer layers (dermis). It is characterized by itching, blisters, redness, swelling, scabbing, and scaly skin. One of the most common types of dermatitis is atopic dermatitis, which is also one of the most common skin conditions in general. In cases of atopic dermatitis skin also becomes drier than normal due to increased water loss from the epidermis. Atopic dermatitis is common in people who suffer from asthma or allergies, such as hay fever. It is especially common in babies and young children. Conventional medical treatments for atopic dermatitis typically use mineral oil lotions or other medicinal ointments, and sometimes oral medications.

Research has found that coconut oil applied topically can be an effective treatment for relieving the symptoms of atopic dermatitis. One such study involved 117 pediatric participants with mild to moderate atopic dermatitis. The degree of their condition was scored before, during, and after the study began using a testing method known as a SCORAD index. Their levels of skin hydration were also measured before, during, and after the study, which ran for eight weeks.

During the course of the study the children were divided into two groups, with the first group treated with mineral oil and the second group treated with virgin coconut oil. At the end of the study the children treated with coconut oil decreased their baseline SCORAD index by 68.23 percent, while the mineral oil group's baseline index was reduced by only 38.13 percent. In addition, 47 percent (28 of 59) of the children in the coconut oil group achieved moderate improvement in their condition and 46 percent (27 children) showed an excellent response. In comparison, in the mineral oil group, 34 percent (20 of 58) of the children showed moderate improvement and only 19 percent (11 children) achieved excellent improvement. The children in the coconut oil group also showed greater improvements in their levels of skin hydration. Based on the results of this study the researchers who conducted it stated that virgin coconut oil is clearly superior to mineral oil for the treatment of atopic dermatitis.

Olive oil is sometimes recommended as a self-care treatment for atopic dermatitis. While olive oil can be helpful for this condition, research has shown that coconut oil is even more effective, including for keeping it from spreading. One study that demonstrated coconut oil's superiority to olive oil for treating atopic dermatitis and halting its spread involved 52 adults with the condition from two outpatient dermatitis clinics.

The study ran for a period of four weeks, during which all of the participants were initially tested using the SCORAD index and screened for the presence and level of *Staphylococcus aureus* (SA), a type of bacteria known to cause and spread atopic dermatitis. Prior to the study beginning, 20 of 26 patients in the coconut oil group were found to be infected by SA, while in the mineral oil group 12 of 26 patients were found to have an SA infection.

During the study all of the 26 participants in one clinic were instructed to apply virgin coconut oil twice a day to the area of their skin surrounding their atopic dermatitis, while all 26 patients in the other clinic applied mineral oil to the surrounding skin area twice a day. At the end of the study, only one (5 percent) of the original 20 participants in the coconut oil group who originally presented with SA infection still showed the presence of SA. By contrast, six (50 percent) of the 12 participants in the mineral oil group with SA infections at the start of the study were still infected. In addition, all of the participants in the coconut oil group demonstrated a greater reduction in their original SCORAD index compared to all of the members in the mineral oil group. The authors of the study wrote that coconut oil's broad-spectrum anti-SA and overall antimicrobial properties is the likely reason why coconut oil is superior to olive oil as a treatment for atopic dermatitis.

Dry, Rough Skin

Due to a variety of factors, skin can become dry, flaky, and rough, especially as we age. Research has shown that coconut oil applied to skin can help prevent this from happening and also reverse such skin conditions.

One type of skin condition is known as xerosis, which is characterized by dry, rough, scaly, flaky, and itchy skin. The conventional medical treatment of xerosis is typically skin creams and moisturizing ointments that contain mineral oils and other ingredients. In a study published in the medical journal *Dermatitis* researchers examined how coconut compared to mineral oil in terms of both oils' effectiveness and safety for treating mild to moderate cases of xerosis.

The study was a randomized, controlled clinical trial involving 34 patients with xerosis on their legs. The participants were divided into two groups. The first group applied mineral oil to their legs twice a day for a period of 14 days, while the second group applied virgin coconut oil twice daily for the same period. During the study period the levels of skin hydration and skin fats were measured in both groups of participants, as was skin pH.

By the end of the study, both groups showed significant improvements in their conditions, including improvements in skin hydration and skin lipid levels. Both the mineral oil and coconut oil were also found to be safe for use. However, it was the participants in the coconut oil group who showed the most improvements in their condition when compared to the mineral oil group.

How to Use Coconut Oil On Your Skin

The first thing to remember should you choose to use coconut oil on your skin is to only use organic, extra virgin coconut oil that is free of any other additives or other ingredients. As with its use on hair and scalp you do not need to use a lot of coconut oil. It is safe to use not only on other areas of your body but also your face and neck.

Start with one teaspoon of coconut oil. If necessary, depending on room temperature, you can warm it up slightly so that if liquefies. Then begin gently rubbing and massaging it onto your skin. As you do so you will find that your skin quickly begins to absorb the coconut oil. If you find that the oil starts to pool on your skin it simply means that this area of skin has reached its saturation point. Should that happen, simply move on to other areas of your skin and repeat the process. For areas of excessively dry, rough, or patchy skin you may need to apply a bit more coconut oil to ensure that it gets fully absorbed into the affected area. Such skin areas may require more than one application of coconut oil per day, as well, before you begin to see results.

Unlike commercial skin creams and lotions, coconut oil is quickly absorbed into skin and does not leave a greasy appearance. Nor does it stain as readily as other oils, creams, and lotions do, making coconut oil an ideal massage oil.

Because of how quickly coconut oil is absorbed by skin, unless you over apply it, in most cases there will not be a need to wash it off. Simply let it be fully absorbed and then go about your day (or night, if you apply it before bedtime). With regular use you will soon begin to experience the same healthy skin benefits that coconut oil has for centuries provided Pacific Islanders and people in other regions were coconuts grow.

CONCLUSION

Now that you know more about the benefits coconut oil can provide for your hair and skin, as well as more about the scientific research that verifies those benefits, I hope that you will consider using coconut oil to better ensure the health of your hair and skin. Should you do so, don't be surprised if after a while people start to compliment you on your healthier, more youthful appearance.

In the next chapter, you will discover how and why coconut oil, and coconut flour, are your best choice for your cooking and baking needs.

11.

Cooking and Baking with Coconut Oil and Coconut Flour

I n this chapter we are going to explore the benefits of cooking and baking with coconut oil, as well as the advantages of using coconut flour over the far more commonly used wheat flour. Let's begin by examining the downsides of using other types of oils for cooking and baking.

HEALTH RISKS OF MOST COOKING OILS

There are a number of major health risks that can occur when using most types of vegetable oils, as well as other substances, such as margarine or shortening products such as Crisco, for cooking and baking. All of these cooking and baking products are highly susceptible to damage caused by heat, light, and oxygen. When used for cooking or baking, they can easily become oxidized, resulting in the formation of harmful free radicals. This is particularly true of most vegetable oils, especially polyunsaturated vegetable oils. These oils, which include canola, corn, flaxseed, sesame, safflower, soybean, and sunflower oils, are extremely fragile and can quickly become oxidized when they are exposed to heat, light, and oxygen.

These oils also contain very high amounts of omega-6 fatty acids which, as you learned in Chapter 3, promote chronic inflammation in the body. Chronic inflammation is now recognized as a primary risk factor for nearly all disease conditions. The pro-inflammatory effects caused by the consumption of polyunsaturated oils are significantly exacerbated by the free radicals that are produced when these oils are heated. In addition, consuming foods that are cooked in polyunsaturated oils will result in oxidized cholesterol being introduced into your bloodstream. This is especially true of canola oil. As you also learned in Chapter 3, oxidized cholesterol, not normal cholesterol itself, is a primary risk factor for heart disease and stroke.

Furthermore, the oxidation process that occurs when vegetable oils are exposed to heat through cooking or baking can also cause the free radicals that are produced to act as carcinogens (cancer-causing agents) in the body. This is one more very important reason why such oils should not be used for cooking or baking.

The main reason that unsaturated (both monounsaturated and polyunsaturated) oils so easily become oxidized and form free radicals has to do with their double carbon bonds, which you also learned about in Chapter 3. These double bonds act as "weak links" in the fatty acids' carbon chains. Heat, light, and oxygen exposure all act to easily damage and break these double carbon bonds. Free radicals are produced when the bonds are broken.

When vegetable oils are used for cooking and baking the free radicals that are produced can cause unhealthy clumping or "stickiness" of blood platelets once the oils are consumed from eating the foods that are cooked or baked in them. Such platelet stickiness can lead to the formation of dangerous blood clots capable of causing heart attacks and stroke. The increased risk of platelet stickiness can also occur when saturated oils composed of long-chain fatty acids (LCFAs) are used for cooking.

In addition to the above health risks caused by the use of vegetable oils for cooking and baking, there is another important disadvantage such oils have. They do not have a long shelf life, even when they are not used for cooking or baking. As a result, if they are not used soon after they are purchased, they can go rancid, resulting in them not only tasting bad, but making them even more unfit for consumption.

Given the dangers to health posed by most vegetable oils, some health experts recommend cooking with olive oil, especially extra virgin olive oil instead. While it is certainly true that olive oil has been shown to reduce the risk of heart disease and other serious health conditions, including breast cancer, because of the healthy amounts of omega-3 oils that it contains, research has also shown that these benefits are greatly reduced when olive oil is heated. In addition, in high cooking temperatures olive oil can also be transformed into a carcinogen; for this reason, olive oil should best be used unheated, such as in salad dressings.

THE COCONUT OIL ADVANTAGE

Now that you know of the dangers posed by cooking with most other types of oils you will want to ensure that the oil you use to prepare cooked foods is one that is healthy. One that does not become oxidized and produce free radicals, does not promote platelet stickiness, and does not increase levels of oxidized cholesterol in the bloodstream. As the cultures of southern India and the Pacific islands have long known, coconut oil is the solution you are looking for. The people in such cultures have used coconut oil for all of their cooking and baking needs for centuries, including for preparing a variety of fried foods, all without ever exhibiting the same levels of degenerative diseases so common in the United States, so long as they also followed their coconut-rich traditional diets. That's because cooking and baking with coconut oil poses none of the health risks associated with vegetable oils, as well as other saturated oils.

The primary reason why this is so is because the medium chain fatty acids (MCFAs) that coconut oil contains are far less susceptible to damage caused by heat, light, and oxygen. Moreover, in comparison to most other types of cooking oils, the fats in coconut oil remain stable when heated and are able to withstand higher temperatures than other oils. As a result, when coconut oil is used for cooking or baking it does not become oxidized and thus does not produce free radicals. In addition, the MCFAs in coconut oil when it is used for cooking or baking do not elevate blood cholesterol levels or cause platelet stickiness. Just as importantly, coconut oil's MCFAs are easily absorbed by the body to quickly supply energy. And the antioxidants that coconut oil contains also help to protect against free radicals that may already be present in the body. And finally, when coconut oil is used for cooking or baking it adds texture to and enhances the taste of foods, making it a delicious cooking and baking choice.

In addition, coconut oil, because of the stability of its MCFAs, has a very long shelf life and can safely be stored for months without the risk of it becoming rancid. This means that, besides retaining its flavor and health-promoting properties far longer than other types of cooking oils, coconut oil can also be a more economical choice when it comes to your cooking and baking needs, making things easier on your wallet. Because of its stability, coconut oil also does not need to be kept refrigerated or placed away from light.

Guidelines for Cooking and Baking With Coconut Oil

You can use coconut oil for cooking or baking exactly as you would use any other type of oil. Simply substitute coconut oil for any other oil used as an ingredient in recipes. The amount of coconut oil to use will be the same as the amount of the other oil called for in the recipes.

Coconut oil can be used for grilling, frying, stir-frying, and other cooking methods, such as scrambling eggs or making omelets, or simply reheating food. It can also be used as a substitute ingredient in recipes calling for butter or cream sauces, such as rice or pasta dishes. Although I do not recommend eating fried foods regularly, when you do choose to fry foods coconut oil is your best option. Unlike other oils, it does not spatter when used to fry foods, nor is it absorbed into foods in the same way that vegetable oils are.

Being part Italian, I have a soft spot in my heart (and stomach) for pasta dishes. Prior to discovering the benefits of coconuts and coconut oil, whenever I boiled pasta to prepare a pasta dish I used to add extra virgin olive oil to water once it came to a boil to prevent the pasta from clumping as it boiled. Even so, I also stirred the pasta regularly to further prevent clumping. Now, I use coconut oil instead, and I find that it prevents clumping of pasta even when I let it boil on the stove unattended. Try this yourself and see.

As you learned earlier in this book, coconut oil remains solid at room temperatures below 76 degree Fahrenheit. Once heated or warmed, however, it will quickly become liquid, making it easy to measure. When in its solid form, its texture is very much like butter, and is in fact sometimes called coconut butter. Once it turns liquid, it has a mild and satisfying taste that adds flavor to the foods it is used to cook or bake.

One other thing to consider when cooking with coconut oil is that it has a moderate smoke point, meaning that when cooking temperatures become too high, coconut oil will start to smoke. Coconut oil's smoke point is higher than most other oils, however, which is another one of its advantages. Smoke point refers to the temperature at which the oil begins to break down and produce free radicals. When coconut oil begins to smoke its healing properties can be destroyed in much the same way that overheating can destroy enzymes found in fruits and vegetables. For best results, cooking temperatures should be kept under 350 degrees Fahrenheit. That's still high enough to cook any type of food, regardless of what cooking method you choose to use. (If your stovetop lacks a temperature gauge you needn't worry. Just be on the lookout for coconut oil to start smoking. If it does so it means the cooking temperature is too high and needs to be reduced until the smoking stops.) For baking purposes, however, you can set the temperature somewhat higher if called for (400 to 450 degrees F) because of how the moisture in the other ingredients in the foods being baked protect against smoking.

If you are new to using coconut oil for cooking or baking, I encourage you to experiment with using it. Once you do so, I think you will find, as I did, that it is ideal for both cooking and baking. Just be sure to choose a brand of organic extra virgin coconut oil that is free of any other ingredients or additives.

THE COCONUT FLOUR ADVANTAGE

In recent years, coconut flour has become known as a healthy alternative to wheat flour. Its rise in popularity is in part due to the fact that, unlike wheat flour, coconut flour does not contain gluten, a combination of proteins that a significant percentage of people today have difficulty tolerating when wheat products (as well as barley, rye, and oat products, all of which also contain gluten) are consumed. Researchers estimate that as much as 50 percent of all people today suffer from some degree of gluten intolerance. Approximately 3 million Americans suffer from celiac disease, an autoimmune condition linked to gluten that can cause serious health problems within the gastrointestinal tract and greatly increase the risk of gastrointestinal cancer.

Coconut flour is produced from the flesh, or "meat," of mature coconuts. The meat is dried and processed after coconut oil is extracted from the meat, and then ground into a powder. In appearance coconut flour is very similar to wheat flour.

In addition to being gluten-free, coconut flour has a number of other health advantages compared to wheat and other types of flour. Nearly 60 percent of coconut flour consists of dietary fiber. This is a higher percentage of dietary fiber than any other type of flour. Fiber is essential for the smooth functioning of the entire gastrointestinal tract, prevents both constipation and diarrhea, and reduces the risk of colon and certain other types of cancer.

Coconut flour also is lower in carbohydrates compared to wheat and other flours, while also relatively high in protein. This combination of low carbohydrates and high fiber makes coconut flour an ideal alternative to wheat and other flours for people wanting to lose weight. Its high fiber content helps promote a feeling of fullness, while its low level of carbohydrates helps to minimize the blood sugar and insulin spikes associated with unhealthy weight gain. In addition, coconut flour also contains all of the vitamins and minerals that you read about in Chapter 2, including calcium, magnesium, phosphorus, potassium, selenium, zinc, and vitamins C, E, B1, B2, B3, B5, B6, and B9. It also contains the fatty acids (MCFAs) found in coconut and coconut oil, providing their healthy benefits as well.

Another important advantage that coconut flour has over other types of flours is that it is produced without being treated with sulfites. Sulfites are sulfur-based preservatives that can cause a variety of health-related problems, including symptoms such as asthma, nasal and sinus congestion, headache, and postnasal drip. Moreover, unlike most wheat and other flours, most coconut flour produced today is organic.

Is Gluten the Problem or Is it Something Else?

Wheat has been a staple food source around the world for many centuries. During most of that time, few people ever experienced health problems from eating wheat products. Until recently, celiac disease was virtually nonexistent and gluten intolerance was also unheard of. It was not until the late 20th century that health issues related to wheat consumption began to appear to any noticeable degree. Since that time, the incidences of both gluten intolerance and celiac disease have continued to increase in each successive decade. Yet, if gluten was not a problem for centuries, why has it become the health hazard it is for so many people today? What has changed?

According to some researchers, most notably, Stephanie Seneff, PhD, a Senior Research Scientist at the Massachusetts Institute of Technology (MIT), the answer to that question lies not in gluten itself. Rather, it can be traced to the introduction of the chemical herbicide glyphosate, more commonly known today by its patented trademarked named Roundup®.

Roundup was first introduced into the marketplace by its developer, the Monsanto corporation, in 1973, and touted as an effective weed and unwanted grass killer. Now that its patent has expired, glyphosate products are today manufactured and sold around the world by multiple chemical companies under more than 30 different trade names. Each year, more than 200 million pounds (100,000 tons) of glyphosate products are used by farmers and agriculture conglomerates in at least 160 countries around the world, including, most especially, the United States. The use of such products has become so prevalent that glyphosate is now found in many of our planet's bodies of water. According to health experts, such as the renowned C. Norman Shealy, it is now a component of over 70 percent of rain water that falls across the United States. Although Monsanto and other manufacturers of glyphosate products continue to claim otherwise, glyphosate is considered by a growing number of researchers to be a risk factor for cancer. In fact, in 2015, scientists from the International Agency for Research on Cancer, the cancer research arm of the World Health Organization, classified glyphosate as a "probable carcinogen." In that same year, California's Environmental Protection Agency (Cal/EPA) listed glyphosate as carcinogenic and now requires Monsanto to include warning labels for Roundup products sold in California stating that it causes cancer.

So what does all of this have to do with wheat and gluten intolerance, you may ask. Quite a bit, according to the research Dr. Seneff has conducted. That's because glyphosate today is used not only to kill weeds and prevent weed growth, it is also widely sprayed onto wheat and other crops, such as cane sugar, prior to the crops being harvested. Doing so dessicates (dries out) wheat and other crops, making it easier for them to be harvested and reducing the wear and tear on the blades of harvesting machines. Nearly all wheat crops grown in the U.S. today are sprayed with Roundup or other glyphosate products prior to being harvested.

The problem with this lies in the fact that once glyphosate is sprayed on wheat and other crops it gets absorbed by the crops and is carried into our bodies when glyphosate-sprayed wheat and wheat products made from such wheat are consumed. Once in the body, glyphosate disrupts the normal pathways that are part of the healthy bacteria in the GI tract, causing these bacteria to die or be damaged. Just as nature has placed a wide array of healthy bacteria in soil in order for vegetation to grow, so too do our bodies rely on healthy gut bacteria in order to stay healthy. Without them, unhealthy bacteria and fungi, such as candida, are able to spread unchecked. Once these healthy bacteria die off or become damaged, a wide array of possible gastrointestinal conditions can arise, which over time can result in a host of other health problems. According to Dr. Seneff and others, while gluten is blamed for such problems, the actual and more harmful culprit is most likely the glyphosate that is carried into the body when wheat is consumed.

Fortunately, coconuts are not sprayed with Roundup or other glyphosate products, and therefore coconut flour does not contain any glyphosate residue. This is one more important reason why choosing to use coconut flour instead of wheat flour is a good idea.

Guidelines for Using Coconut Flour

Coconut flour can be used to bake a variety of breads, cakes, and other baked goods. However, when using coconut flour for baking there are a number of things you must consider. First, you cannot simply substitute coconut flour for wheat or other flours in a 1:1 ratio. The reasons for this are twofold. The first reason has to do with the fact that coconut flour is gluten-free. Gluten is what gives dough its elastic texture and holds it together. Coconut flour by itself will not hold dough together.

In addition, coconut flour is much more absorbent than wheat and other flours. For this reason, most baking recipes for which coconut flour is an ingredient call for using far less coconut flour than the same recipes that use wheat flour instead. Typically, baking with coconut flour only requires $1/4$ cup to $1/3$ cup of coconut flour in place of one cup of wheat or other flours. In addition, coconut flour baking recipes usually call for a large number of eggs to be used, due to the flour's high absorption factor. The eggs help to provide texture to cakes, breads, and other baked goods made from coconut flour, and to hold them together and keep them from becoming too dry. (Coconut flour also tends to be more dense and drier than wheat and other flours.)

As a general rule, for every cup of coconut flour used you will also need to include six beaten eggs. For added moisture and consistency, also add one cup of liquid. Many recipes recommend the liquid be coconut milk. Because of the amount of eggs used, along with coconut flour's own protein content, baked goods made from coconut flour supply more protein than other baked goods, with far less carbohydrates; another reason why baking with coconut flour is a healthier option than baking with wheat flour. Because coconut flour contains its own supply of natural sugars, there usually is no need to add sugar or other sweeteners to the baked goods. Instead, coconut flour will provide its own slightly sweet flavor to what you choose to bake.

When first beginning to bake using coconut flour it is best to rely on proven coconut flour recipes before you start to experiment on your own. Providing such recipes is beyond the scope of this book, but you can find them online. Books about baking with coconut flour are also available.

You can also obtain the benefits of coconut flour without baking. Simply add the flour to smoothies to create delicious, protein-rich drinks. You can also use coconut flour to thicken soups, sauces, and curries, as is traditionally done in cultures around the world where coconuts are a staple food.

CONCLUSION

Now that you know more about how and why coconut oil is a superior cooking choice compared to other oils, as well as the advantages coconut flour offers over wheat and other types of flour, I hope that you will apply what you have learned in this chapter whenever oil or flour is called for in cooking or baking recipes. By using coconut oil and coconut flour, you will be taking another step in achieving and maintaining better health.

12.

Guidelines for Buying and Using Coconuts and Coconut Products

Coconuts are available in nearly all grocery stores across the United States today, and many grocery and health food stores also carry coconut oil, coconut milk, and coconut water. What follows are guidelines to help you get the most benefits from coconuts and coconut products.

WHOLE COCONUTS

Coconuts are typically found in the produce section of grocery stores. When purchasing them it is important that you make sure they are fresh, not overripe. This is difficult to do from relying on their appearance alone. Coconuts can remain fresh for many weeks after they are harvested. The fresher they are, the more liquid they contain inside.

Choosing a Fresh Coconut

To determine if a coconut is fresh or not, pick it up and shake it. You will be able to hear the liquid sloshing around inside fresh coconuts when they are shaken. With overripe coconuts, the amount of liquid will be minimal. If you don't easily hear the sound of sloshing liquid, put it back.

Another thing to look for is the condition of the coconut's "eyes." Coconuts have three "eyes," or indentations. Before purchasing coconuts, inspect the eyes to ensure that they are completely intact. You want to avoid buying coconuts if the eyes appear to have cracks or show signs of mold on and around them.

Opening the Coconut

Once you have selected your coconuts and brought them home, the next step of course is opening them.

- The first step in this process is to drain the coconut. To do this, examine each of the 3 eyes or indentations. Usually you will find that one of them is softer or weaker than the other two. Once you find it, use a sharp, thin knife, metal skewer, or a screwdriver to puncture the eye, creating a hole.

- Then place the coconut over a bowl (I prefer a measuring cup, on top of which most coconuts can easily rest without being held) and let the liquid inside the coconut drain into it. Be sure to let the liquid completely drain. Typically this can take a few minutes and you may need to shake the coconut from time to time to ensure that all of the liquid drains out. Fresh coconuts usually contain between one-half to three-fourths of a cup of liquid. This is the coconut water, which you can drink or set aside to use for cooking, baking, or flavoring of foods. (I prefer to simply drink it, finding the taste delicious and refreshing.)

- Once the coconut is completely drained it is ready to be opened. Because of the hardness of its shell, you will need a hammer or mallet to crack the shell. I recommend covering the bottom half of the coconut with a folded towel or thick paper towels and then setting it atop of your kitchen counter or another hard surface. Then use a mallet or hammer to strike along the exposed shell until the coconut cracks. You may have to use some force in order to succeed at this. You want to turn the coconut as you strike so that it begins to crack in half. Once it does so, you can pry it completely in half with your fingers.

- Once the coconut splits in half, set both halves face down on a plate and use your mallet or hammer to tap along the sides of the shell. This will help loosen up the coconut flesh, or meat, inside.

- Once the flesh is loosened, wedge a butter knife between the flesh and the shell to pry the flesh away from the shell until it is completely separated. When separating the flesh from the shell, you will find a thin, brown, fibrous skin on the outside of the flesh. This is what connected the flesh to the shell. You can use a vegetable peeler to remove this skin, leaving the flesh of the coconut ready to eat. If you don't eat the flesh immediately, be sure to refrigerate it and eat or cook with it within a few days. Otherwise it will spoil.

Of course, you can avoid this entire process simply by purchasing already dried and shredded coconut at your local grocery store. Dried, shredded coconut contains the same amount of nutrients found in fresh coconut, including coconut's medium-chain fatty acids. Besides being a much more convenient alternative to having to go through the process of cracking opening fresh coconuts, dried, shredded coconut is more resistant to spoilage and oxidation. Even so, be sure to check the expiration date when purchasing packaged shredded coconut.

COCONUT WATER

As mentioned above, the average fresh mature coconut contains between one-half and three-fourths of a cup of coconut water. If you want the freshest and most nutritious coconut water, however, you need to choose fresh, young coconuts. As you learned in Chapter 7, these coconuts are unlike the riper, brown coconuts commonly found in the produce section of grocery stores. Instead, if your grocery or local health food store carries them, they will be found in the store's refrigerated section because they are highly perishable. To obtain the water, simply puncture the young coconut just as you would do with coconuts sold in the produce section.

The downside of this approach is that young coconuts, like their older, unrefrigerated brown counterparts, do not supply much coconut water in terms of content. For this reason, commercial bottled coconut water products can now be readily found in most grocery and health food stores in the U.S. But, as I also pointed out in Chapter 7, commercial bottled coconut water is not as healthy as coconut water derived from fresh coconuts because its nutritional content is not as fresh and often further diminished in potency due to being processed and pasteurized. In addition, many coconut water products contain reconstituted concentrates of coconut water. In order to produce such concentrates, coconut water first needs to be heated and then reduced into a syrup, which is later reconstituted with water prior to being bottled or otherwise packaged. This method saves on production costs, yet the heating process also destroys much of the coconut water's nutrient content.

A number of commercial brands of coconut water also contain added sugar. Sugar is unhealthy and should be avoided. If you enjoy drinking bottled coconut water, be sure to check the label to see if the product is made from concentrate, pasteurized, and/or contains sugar, preservatives, or other additives. If it does, I recommend you avoid the product.

For a list of certified organic coconut water products, see the Resources section on page 177.

COCONUT MILK

As I mentioned in this book's Introduction, although the terms are often used interchangeably, coconut milk and coconut water are not the same thing. Coconut water in its purest form refers to the liquid that is found inside coconuts. Coconut milk, by contrast, is produced by combining the meat of the coconut with water.

Today there are a number of coconut milk products that are commonly available in grocery and health food stores across the United States. Not all of them are the same, and knowing the difference is vitally important when it comes to your health. When you are considering purchasing coconut milk always check the label.

Many coconut milk products contain a variety of unhealthy additives that you want to avoid. Among them are dietary emulsifiers, which act as thickening agents and keep ingredients from separating. One of the most common emulsifiers found in commercial coconut milk products is carrageenan. It is known to cause digestive and other gastrointestinal problems. It has been linked to obesity, pre-diabetes and diabetes, metabolic syndrome, colitis, and other inflammatory bowel diseases because of the way that it disrupts the balance of healthy bacteria in the gastrointestinal tract.

Other commonly found additives include guar gum or locust bean gum. These can cause bloating, flatulence, and other digestive problems. Corn dextrin and/or xanthum gum, both of which are commonly derived from genetically-modified corn, can also cause gastrintestinal problems. Added sugar and/or so-called natural flavors, are other common additives and are also unhealthy and also unnecessary, since there is no need to sweeten coconut milk.

The healthiest coconut milk products are typically sold in cans and contain only coconut oil. However, many canned items today are treated with bisphenol A (BPA), as are many containers made from plastic. BPA mimics the hormone estrogen and has been linked to a long list of serious health conditions, including cancer, diabetes, and obesity because of the way BPA acts both as a toxin in the body, and a disruptor of the body's overall endocrine (hormone) system. Fortunately, a number of manufacturers are now eliminating BPA from metal and plastic containers. So look for coconut milk that is both free of other additives and sold in containers that are BPA-free. (*See* Resources on page 177.)

If you prefer, you can also make your own healthy coconut milk at home. All that is required is dried, shredded coconut, pure, filtered water, a blender, and a wire mesh strainer. In your blender, combine the shredded coconut and water in a 1:2 ratio (for example, 4 cups of shredded coconut to 8 cups of pure, filtered water). Then blend at a high speed for one to two minutes. Once both ingredients are fully blended, separate out any remaining coconut pulp by pushing the mixture through a strainer placed over a glass bottle or bowl. (Rather than discarding the remaining pulp, I prefer to eat it either by itself or mixed with organic yogurt.)

Whether you buy or make your own coconut milk, you can use it as a drink on its own or added to a smoothie, pour it on cereal as a healthy alternative to dairy milk, and use it for cooking or baking. Keep unused portions refrigerated.

COCONUT OIL

Many people, including me, prefer to obtain the health benefits of coconuts primarily from coconut oil. I use coconut oil for all of my cooking needs, and also frequently take one to two tablespoons of coconut oil as a nutritional supplement during the day to help provide my body with the healthy fatty acids (MCFAs) and other nutrients that coconut oil contains.

You can find my recommendations for how to cook and bake with coconut oil in Chapter 11. To briefly recap, coconut oil can be used as a substitute for any other type of vegetable oil when used for cooking. For more on how to use coconut oil for both cooking and baking purposes, see *Guidelines For Cooking and Baking With Coconut Oil,* beginning on page 159.

To use coconut oil as a nutritional supplement, begin slowly and take no more than one tablespoon per day. Doing so will help your body get used to consuming raw coconut oil and minimize any intestinal discomfort that consumption of coconut oil can sometimes initially cause until your body grows accustomed to it. Most people only require a tablespoon or two of coconut oil a day to obtain an adequate supply of healthy medium-chain fatty acids, but coconut oil is safe to consume at higher doses (up to four to eight tablespoons per day). However, if you choose to consume coconut oil at a higher level, it is best if you consume it in doses that are divided throughout the day.

I prefer to simply take one or two spoonfuls of coconut oil by itself. Many people prefer instead to mix it in foods, such as yogurt, or in beverages, such as almond milk or as an addition to homemade coconut milk. Coconut oil can also be added to smoothies and even juices such as orange juice. You can also use it to make a healthy alternative to mayonnaise. (See page 172.)

Be sure that you only use pure, extra virgin organic coconut oil, with no other additives. You do not want to use any other type of coconut oil because nonorganic, refined, or otherwise processed coconut oil can be bleached, excessively heated, and/or otherwise chemically processed in order to increase its shelf-life. Processing coconut oil to any degree alters its chemical makeup, including the chemical makeup of the MCFAs coconut oil contains, making them unfit for human consumption.

If you choose to add a tablespoon or more of coconut oil to your daily health regimen, you should also be sure to increase your daily consumption of both raw and fermented vegetables. That's because MCFAs contained in

Using Coconut Oil to Make a Healthy Alternative to Mayonnaise

Most commercial brands of mayonnaise are loaded with unhealthy oils, especially canola oil and/or corn or soybean oils, many of which are also derived from genetically modified corn and soybeans. Even many health food brands of mayonnaise contain canola oil or else swap it out for other vegetable oils such as safflower oil. In addition, many brands of store-bought mayonnaise—both commercial and health food brands—also contain sugar and other unhealthy additives.

Here is an easy recipe you can follow to make healthy coconut mayonnaise. The ingredients you will need are:

- Two raw eggs (ideally from a free-range hen)

- One to two tablespoons or raw, organic, nonpasteurized apple cider vinegar with "the mother" (check the label)

- A dash of sea salt (no more than a quarter teaspoon)

- One and a half cups of organic coconut oil (remember, coconut oil turns solid in temperatures below 76 degree Fahrenheit; if necessary, liquify the coconut oil first using a low heat).

Combine the first three ingredients above plus half of a cup of liquid coconut oil in a blender and blend together for one minute. Then, as you continue to run the blender, slowly add the remaining coconut oil to the mixture. Do not add in the rest of the coconut oil all at once. You need to add it slowly in order to achieve the right texture and consistency.

For a zestier version of this recipe, you can also add spices, such as a dash of paprika and/or one or two teaspoons of mustard.

To increase the supply of healthy fats, you can also consider adding half of a medium-sized avocado.

Although homemade coconut mayonnaise can be refrigerated after it is produced, it is best that it be used soon after you make it because the refrigeration process will cause it to solidify, after which it will need to be liquified under a low heat. Usually, heating refrigerated coconut mayonnaise will also affect its texture and consistency. For best results, experiment with the ingredients you use to satisfy your taste buds, and make only as much of this healthy mayonnaise alternative as you intend to use at one time.

uncooked coconut oil, especially lauric acid, have been show to transport a certain class of substances known as lipopolysaccharides out of the gastrointestinal tract and into the bloodstream. Once there, lipopolysaccharides can act as toxins in the body. Eating raw, green and other nonstarchy vegetables, as well as fermented vegetables, such as sauerkraut, can help keep lipopolysaccharides within the GI tract, where they belong. The ability of such vegetables to do this is due to the fact that, once they are digested, they produce various types of healthy acids in the GI tract that act as checks on lipopolysaccharides.

Overall, however, coconut oil is perfectly safe for most people to use. The key, as mentioned, is to start slowly if you are unused to consuming it and to pay attention to how you feel as you consume it.

CONCLUSION

By following the above suggestions and guidelines you can easily start to make the inclusion of coconuts and its various products a part of a healthy diet and overall daily health routine. By doing so, you will soon begin to notice the difference coconuts can make for your health as you begin to obtain the many important health benefits coconut and its milk, water, and oil can provide.

Conclusion

Now that you have read this far you know why coconut, along with its milk, water, oil, and flour, are so prized by people all around the globe who live in lands where coconuts grow and are a staple part of their traditional diets. More importantly, you now know of the many important health benefits that coconuts and the milk, water, oil, and flour that are derived from them can provide you and your loved ones.

What you do with the knowledge you have gained from reading this book is, of course, up to you. My hope is that you will put it to good use by applying what you have learned. I encourage you to experiment. The next time you are in your local grocery or health food store, consider purchasing a raw coconut or else a supply of packaged, dried, shredded coconut. See what happens when you substitute extra virgin coconut oil for other oils when you cook and bake. Try making your own homemade coconut milk or coconut mayonnaise by following the recipes I shared with you in chapters 11 and 12. See what happens when you swap out wheat flour for coconut flour the next time you bake.

Remember: The only way that you will know for sure if coconut and its milk, water, oil, and flour can improve your health is to begin using them on a regular basis. If you are willing to do so, and also willing to follow an overall healthy diet and lifestyle, I think you will soon find that coconuts are a delicious way of helping to ensure your good health.

Thank you very much for reading this book. I greatly appreciate you for taking the time to do so. Now put what you have learned to good use.

Health and Blessings!

Resources

Today, you can find coconuts, extra virgin coconut oil, coconut milk, coconut flour, and other coconut products in most grocery and health food stores across the United States. The following companies also supply high quality, organic coconut oil, flour, and other coconut products. Look for them at your local grocery and health food stores. Or you can order them directly from the companies' websites. The products they supply are also available at Amazon.com.

Artisana Organics
810 81st Avenue, Suite B
Oakland, CA 94621
(866) 237-8688
www.artisanaorganics.com
Supplier of coconut oil and coconut butter.

Coconut Oil Online
(800) 922-1744
www.coconutoil-online.com
Supplier of coconut oil, coconut cream, and dried, shredded coconut sold under various brand names.

Edward and Sons Trading Company
P.O. Box 1326
Carpinteria, CA 93014
(805) 684-8500
www.edwardandsons.com

Supplier of coconut cream, coconut milk, coconut flour, coconut flakes, and dried, shredded coconut sold under the brand name Let's Do Organic.

Healthy Traditions
PO Box 333
Springville, CA 93265
www.healthytraditions.com
Supplier of coconut oil, coconut flour, coconut cream, and dried, shredded coconut sold under the brand name Tropical Traditions.

Natural Value Products
14 Waterthrush Ct
Sacramento, CA 95831
(916) 836-3561
www.naturalvalue.com
Supplier of coconut cream and coconut milk sold in BPA-free cans.

Nutiva

213 West Cutting Blvd
Richmond, CA 94804
(800) 993-4367
www.nutiva.com
Supplier of coconut oil, coconut flour and other coconut products. Nutiva, provides both organic virgin and organic refined coconut oils. Choose the organic virgin product.

Radiant Life

5277 Aero Drive
Santa Rosa, CA 95403
(888) 593-8333
www.radiantlifecatalog.com
Supplier of coconut oil, coconut flour, and other coconut products.

References

Chapter 1

Gunn BF, Baudouin L, Olsen KM (2011) "Independent Origins of Cultivated Coconut (*Cocos nucifera* L.) in the Old World Tropics." *PLoS ONE* 6(6): e21143.

Harries HC. "The evolution, dissemination and classification of *Cocos nucifera L.*" *Bot. Rev.*44:265–319.

Lebrun P et al, editors. "Coconut. Genetic Diversity of cultivated tropical plants." 2003. Paris, France: Science Publishers Inc and CIRAD, France; 219–238.

MO63.4852. Coconut shell paperweight with PT109 rescue message. John F. Kennedy Presidential Library and Museum. www.jfklibrary.org/Asset-Viewer/Ey5l-6Vagyk2dwA6BTctDZg.aspx

Shipwrecked John F Kennedy Finds Solomon Islanders. World War Two Today. http://ww2today.com/5th-august-1943-shipwrecked-john-f-kennedy-meets-soloman-island-natives

Society for Experimental Biology. "Coconuts could inspire new designs for earthquake-proof buildings." *ScienceDaily.* 5 July 2016.

The Voyage of Magellan: The Journal of Antonio Pigafetta. Prentice-Hall. 1969.

Chapter 2

Kaunitz H. "Nutritional properties of coconut oil." *APCC Quarterly Supplement* 30 Dec 1971:35–37.

Chapter 3

Ahrens EH Jr., et al."Effect on human serum lipids of substituting plant for animal fat in diet." *Proc Soc Exp Biol Med.* 1954;86(4):872–878.

Banneberg G, Serhan CN. "Specialized pro-resolving lipid mediators in the inflammatory response: An update." *Biochim Biopys Acta.* 2010; 1801(12):1260–1273.

Brown MJ, Ferruzzi MG, et al. "Carotenoid bioavailability is higher from salads ingested with full-fat than with fat-reduced salad dressings as measured with electrochemical detection." *Am J Clin Nutr.* 2004;80(2):396–403.

Burr GO, Burr MM. "A New Deficiency Disease Produced by the Rigid Exclusion of Fat From the Diet." *J Biol Chem.* 1929;LXXXII(2):345–367.

Dayton S, et al. "Vitamin E Status of Humans During Prolonged Feeding of Unsaturated Fats." *J Lab Clin Med.* 1965;65:739–747.

Dietary fat and its relation to heart attacks and strokes: Report by the Central Committee for Medical and Community Program of the AHA. 1961;23:133–136.

Feinman RD. "Saturated Fat and Health: Recent Advances in Research." *Lipids.* 2010 Oct; 45(10): 891–892.

Guyenet SJ and Carlson SE. "Increase in Adipose Tissue Linoleic Acid of US Adults in the Last Half Century." *Adv Nutr.* 2015;6:660–664.

Hulbert AJ. "On the importance of fatty acid composition of membranes for aging." *J Theor Biol.* 2005 May 21;234(2):277–88.

Keys A. "Atherosclerosis: a problem in newer public health." *J Mt Sinai Hosp NY.* 1953;20(2):118–139.

Kinsell LW, et al. "Dietary modification of serum cholesterol and phospholipid levels." *J Clin Endocrinol. Metab.* 1952;12(7):909–913.

Kris-Etherton PM et al. "Polyunsaturated fatty acids in the food chain in the United States." *Am J Clin Nutr.* 2000 Jan71(1):179S–188S.

Malhotra A, Redberg RF, Meier P. "Saturated fat does not clog the arteries: coronary heart disease is a chronic inflammatory condition, the risk of which can be effectively reduced from healthy lifestyle interventions." *British Journal of Sports Medicine.* 2017.

Page IH, et al. "Atherosclerosis and the Fat Content of the Diet." *Circulation.* 1957;16:163–178.

Pearce ML and Dayton S. "Incidence of Cancer in Men on a Diet High in Polyunsaturated Fat." *Lancet.* 1971;297(7697):464–467.

Simopoulos AP. "The importance of the ratio of omega-6/omega-3 essential fatty acids." *Biomed Pharmacother.* 2002 Oct;56(8):365–379.

The Lipid Research Clinics Coronary Primary Prevention Trial results. II. "The relationship of coronary heart disease to cholesterol lowering." *JAMA.* 1984;251(3):365–374.

Turpeinen O. "Further Studies on the Unsaturated Fatty Acids Essential in Nutrition." *J Nutr.* 1938;15(4):351–366.

USDA Agricultural Research Service. What We Eat in America, *NHANES* 2007–2008. Table 5. Energy Intakes: Percentages of Energy from Protein, Carbohydrate, Fat, and Alcohol, by Gender and Age, in the United States, 2007–2008.

Available at https://www.ars.usda.gov/ARSUserFiles/80400530/pdf/0708/Table_5_EIN_GEN_07.pdf

U.S. Department of Agriculture, U.S. Department of Health and Human Services. *Dietary Guidelines for Americans 2015–2020.* Available at www.dietaryguidelines.gov.

Yam D, Eliraz A, Berry EM. "Diet and disease—the Israeli paradox: possible dangers of a high omega-6 polyunsaturated fatty acid diet." *Isr J Med Sci.* 1996 Nov;32(11):1134–1143.

Chapter 4

American Heart Association's *Heart Disease and Stroke Statistics—2012 Update.*

Bierenbaum ML, et al. "Modified-fat dietary management of the young male with CD." A five-year report. *JAMA.* Dec 25 1967;202(13):1119–1123.

Bierenbaum ML, et al. "Ten-year experience of modified-fat diets on younger men with coronary heart disease." *Lancet.* 1973;1(7817):1404–1407.

Boscarino J, Erlich PM, Hoffman SN. "Low serum cholesterol and external-cause mortality: Potential implications for research and surveillance." *J Psychiatr Res.* 2009;43(9):848–854.

Cardosa DA et al. "A Coconut Extra Virgin Oil-Rich Diet Increases HDL Cholesterol And Decreases Waist Circumference And Body Mass In Coronary Artery Disease Patients." *Nutr Hosp.* 2015 Nov 1;32(5):2144–2152.

Chakrabarti S, Ramsden CE, et al. "Re-evaluation of the traditional diet-heart hypothesis: analysis of recovered data from Minnesota coronary experiment (1968–73)." *BMJ* 2016;353:i1246.doi:10.1136/bmj.i1246

"Controlled trial of soya-bean oil in myocardial infarction." *Lancet.* Sep 28 1968;2(7570):693–699.

Coronary Heart Disease: The Dietary Sense and Nonsense edited by Dr. George V. Mann, M.D., New York:Veritas Society, 1993.

Dayton S et al. "A Controlled Clinical Trial of a Diet High in Unsaturated Fat in Preventing Complications of Atherosclerosis." *Circulation* 1 July 1969;40:II-1-II-63.

Dreon DM et al. "Change in dietary fat intake is correlated with change in mass of large low-density-lipoprotein particles in men." *Amer J Clin Nutr.* May1998;67(5): 828–836.

de Souza RJ, Mente A, Maroleanu A, et al. "Intake of saturated and trans unsaturated fatty acids and risk of all cause mortality, cardiovascular disease, and type 2 diabetes: systematic review and meta-analysis of observational studies." *BMJ* 2015;351:h3978.doi:10.1136/bmj.h3978

Frantz ID, Jr., et al. "Test of effect of lipid lowering by diet on cardiovascular risk." Minnesota Coronary Survey. *Arteriosclerosis.* Jan-Feb 1989;9(1):129–135.

Guasch-Ferre M et al. "Dietary fat intake and risk of cardiovascular disease and all-cause mortality in a population at high risk of cardiovascular disease." *Amer J Clin Nutr.* December 2015;102(6):1563–1573.

Harris WS, et al. "Omega-6 fatty acids and risk for cardiovascular disease: a science advisory from the AHA Nutrition Subcommittee of the Council on Nutrition,

Physical Activity, and Metabolism; Council on Cardiovascular Nursing; and Council on Epidemiology and Prevention." *Circulation.* 2009;119(6):902–907.

Kummerow FA. "Interaction between sphingomyelin and oxysterols contributes to atherosclerosis and sudden death." *Am J CardiovascDis.* 2013; 3(1): 17–26.

Law MR, Thompson SG, Wald NJ. "Assessing possible hazards of reducing serum cholesterol." *BMJ.* 1994 Feb 5;308(6925):373–379.

Lindeberg S, et al. "Age relations of cardiovascular risk factors in a traditional Melanesian society: the Kitava study." *Am J Clin Nutr.* 1997;66(4):845–852.

Lindeberg S, Lundh B. "Apparent absence of stroke and ischaemic heart disease in a traditional Melanesian island: a clinical study in Kitava." *J Intern Med* 1993 Mar;233(3):269–275.

Lindeberg S et al. "Cardiovascular risk factors in a Melanesian population apparently free from stroke and ischaemic heart disease: the Kitava study." *J Intern Med* 1994 Sep;236(3):331–340.

Malhotra A. "The whole truth about coronary stents: the elephant in the room." *JAMA Intern Med* 2014;174:1367–8.doi:10.1001/jamainternmed.2013.9190.

Morgan RE et al. "Plasma cholesterol and depressive symptoms in older men." *The Lancet.* 1993;341(8837):75–79.

Mozaffarian D, Rimm EB, Herrington DM. "Dietary fats, carbohydrate, and progression of coronary atherosclerosis in postmenopausal women." *Am J Clin Nutr* 2004;80:1175–1184.

Mozaffarian, D and Ludwig, D.S. "The 2015 US Dietary Guidelines: Lifting the Ban on Total Dietary Fat." *Journal of the American Medical Association,* 2015;313(24):2421–2422.

Muller H et al. "A diet rich in coconut oil reduces diurnal postprandial variations in circulating tissue plasminogen activator antigen and fasting lipoprotein (a) compared with a diet rich in unsaturated fat in women." *J. Nutr.* 2003 Nov;133(11):3422–3427.

Petrusson H et al. "Is the use of cholesterol in mortality risk algorithms in clinical guidelines valid? Ten years prospective data from the Norwegian HUNT 2 study." *J of the Eval of Clin Pract.* 2012:18(1):159–168.

Prior IA, et al. "Cholesterol, coconuts, and diet on Polynesian atolls: a natural experiment: the Pukapuka and Tokelau island studies." *Am J Clin Nutr.* 1981;34(8): 1552–1561.

Ramsen CE et al. "Re-evaluation of the traditional diet-heart hypothesis: analysis of recovered data from Minnesota Coronary Experiment (1968–73)." *BMJ* 12 April 2016;353:i1246.

Ravnskov U, et al. "Lack of an association or an inverse association between low-density-lipoprotein cholesterol and mortality in the elderly: a systematic review." *BMJ Open* 2016;6:e010401.doi:10.1136/bmjopen-2015–010401

Ravnskov U et al. "The Questionable Benefits of Exchanging Saturated Fat With Polyunsaturated Fat." *Mayo Clinic Proceedings.* April 2014;89(4):451–453.

Rose GA, et al. "Corn oil in treatment of ischaemic heart disease." *Br Med J.* Jun 12 1965;1(5449):1531–1533.

Rothberg MB. "Coronary artery disease as clogged pipes: a misconceptual model." *Circ Cardiovasc Qual Outcomes* 2013;6:129–32.doi:10.1161/CIRCOUTCOMES.112.967778

Schwingshackl L, Hoffmann G. "Dietary fatty acids in the secondary prevention of coronary heart disease: a systematic review, meta-analysis and meta-regression." *BMJ Open* 2014;4:e004487.

Siri-Tarino PW, Sun Q, Hu FB, Kraus RM. "Meta-analysis of prospective cohort studies evaluating the association of saturated fat with cardiovascular disease." *Am J Clin Nutr.* 2010;91:535–546.

Srivastava RA. "Saturated fatty acid, but not cholesterol, regulates apolipoprotein AI gene expression by posttranscriptional mechanism." *Biochem Mol Biol.* Sep 1994;34(2):393–402.

Taubes, Gary. *Vegetable oils, (Francis) Bacon, Bing Crosby, and the American Heart Association.* July 17, 2017. http://garytaubes.com/vegetable-oils-francis-bacon-bing -crosby-and-the-american-heart-association

Chapter 5

Costantini LC, Barr LJ, Vogel JL, Henderson ST. "Hypometaolism as a therapeutic target in Alzheimer's disease." *BMC Neurosci.* 2008;9 Suppl 2:S16.

Henderson ST. "High carbohydrate diets and Alzheimer's disease." *Medical Hypotheses.* May 2004, 62(5):689–700.

Henderson ST. "Ketone Bodies as a Therapeutic for Alzheimer's Disease." *Neurotherapeutics.* 2008; 5(3):470–80.

Henderson ST et al. "Study of the ketogenic agent AC-1202 in mild to moderate Alzheimer's disease: a randomized, double-blind, placebo-controlled, multicenter trial." Nutr Metab (Lond). 2009;6: 31.

Nafar F, Mearow KM. "Coconut Oil Attenuates the Effects of Amyloid-[beta] on Cortical Neurons In Vitro." *J. Alzheimers Dis.* 2014;39(2):233.7.

Newport, Mary MD. *Alzheimer's Disease: What If There Was a Cure?* Basic Health Publications. Laguna Beach, CA: 2011.

Newport, Mary MD. Interview with Dr. Mary T. Newport. https:/blog.bulletproof. com/wp-content/uploads/2014/07/Transcript-13-Mary-Newport.pdf.

Reger MA, Henderson ST et al., "Effects of beta-hydroxybutyrate on cognition in memory-impaired adults." *Neurobiol Aging.* 2004 Mar;25(3):311–314.

Wlaz P, Socala K, et al. "Anticon- 297 vulsant profile of caprylic acid, a main constituent of the 298 medium-chain triglyceride (MCT) ketogenic diet in mice." *Neuropharmacology* 2012:62(4), 1882–1889.

Zhao, W, Varghese, M, et al. (2012). "Caprylic Triglyceride as a Novel Therapeutic

Approach to Effectively Improve the Performance and Attenuate the Symptoms Due to the Motor Neuron Loss in ALS Disease." *Plos ONE*, 7(11), e49191.

Chapter 6

Dayrit, Conrado. *Coconut Oil In Health And Disease: Its And Monolaurin's Potential As Cure For Hiv/Aids.* Available at http://www.coconutoil.com/Dayrit.pdf

Enig, MG: *Coconut Oil: An Anti-bacterial, Anti-viral Ingredient for Food,* Nutrition and Health. AVOC Lauric Symposium. Manila, Philippines Oct. 17, 1997.

Hierholzer, J.C. and Kabara J.J. "In vitro effects on Monolaurin compounds on enveloped RNA and DNA viruses." *J. Food Safety* 1982;4:1–12.

Issacs, C.E. et al. "Inactivation of enveloped viruses in human bodily fluids by purified lipids." *Annals of the New York Academy of Sciences* 1994;724:457–464.

Kabara, J.J. "Antimicrobial agents derived from fatty acids." *Journal of the American Oil Chemists Society* 1984;61:397–403.

Kabara, JJ. "Fatty Acids and Derivatives as Antimicrobial Agents - A Review - Symposium on the Pharmacological Effects of Lipids." Edited by JJ Kabara, *AOCS* p. 1–13. 1978.

Chapter 7

Alleyne T et al. "The control of hypertension by use of coconut water and mauby: two tropical food drinks." *West Indian Med J.* 2005 Jan;54(1):3–8.

Alves NF, de Queiroz TM, et al. "Acute Treatment with Lauric Acid Reduces Blood Pressure and Oxidative Stress in Spontaneously Hyptertensive Rats." *Basic Clin Pharmacol Toxicol.* 2017 Apr;120(4):348–353.

Alves NF, Porpino K, Monteiro M, Gomes E, Braga V. "Coconut oil supplementation and physical exercise improves baroreflex sensitivity and oxidative stress in hypertensive rats." *Applied Physiology, Nutrition, and Metabolism.* 2015. 40(4): 393–400.

Galitzer, Michael and Trivieri, Larry Jr. *Outstanding Health: The 6 Essential Keys To Maximize Your Energy and Well Being.* Los Angeles CA: AHA Publishing. 2015.

Ismail I, Singh R, Sirisinghe RG. "Rehydration with sodium-enriched coconut water after exercise-induced dehydration." *Southeast Asian J Trop Med Public Health.* 2007 Jul;38(4):769–785.

Chapter 8

Assuncao ML et al. "Effects of dietary coconut oil on the biochemical and anthropometric profiles of women presenting abdominal obesity." *Lipids.* 2009 Jul;44(7):593–601.

Dullo AG et al. "Twenty-four-hour energy expenditure and urinary catecholamines of humans consuming low-to-moderate amounts of medium-chain triglycerides: A dose-response study in a human respiratory chamber." *Eur. J. Clin. Nutr.* Mar 1996. 50(3):152–158.

Liau KM et al. "An Open-Label Pilot Study to Assess the Efficacy and Safety of Virgin Coconut Oil in Reducing Visceral Adiposity." *ISRN Pharmacol.* 2011 Mar 15; Volume 2011, Article ID 949686, 7 pages. doi:10.5402/2011/949686.

Lindeberg S et al. "Low serum insulin in traditional Pacific Islanders-the Kitiva Study." *Metabolism* 1999;48(10):1216–1219.

O'Donnell J, Barry E, Covington K. "Obesity, inactivity could outpace smoking in cancer death risk." *USA Today.* June 9, 2017.

Pittet PG, Halliday D, Bateman PE. "Site differences in the fatty acid composition of subcutaneous adipose tissue of obese women." *Br J Nutr.* 1979 Jul;42(1):57–61.

Scalfi L et al. "Postprandial thermogenesis in lean and obese subjects after meals supplemented with medium-chain and long-chain triglycerides." *Amer J Clin Nutr.* May 1991. 53(5):1130–1133.

Stanhope JM, Prior IA. "The Tokelau island migrant study: prevalence and incidence of diabetes mellitus." *NZ Med J.* Dec 10, 1980;92(673):417–421.

St-Onge M-P et al. "Impact of medium and long chain triglycerides consumption on appetite and food intake in overweight men." *Eur J of Clin Nutrition.* Oct 2014.68:1134–1140.

St-Onge M-P, Jones PJH. "Physiological Effects of Medium-Chain Triglycerides: Potential Agents in the Prevention of Obesity." *J. Nutr.* March 1, 2002. 132(3): 329–332.

Stubbs RJ, Habron CG. "Covert manipulation of the ratio of medium- to long-chain triglycerides in isoenergetically dense diets: Effect on food intake in ad libitum feeding men." *International J of Obesity* June 1996. 20(5):435–44.

"The GBD 2015 Obesity Collaborators. Health Effects of Overweight and Obesity in 195 Countries over 25 years." *New Eng J. Med.* June 12, 2017.

Chapter 9

Asokan S et al. "Effect of oil pulling on halitosis and microorganisms causing halitosis: a randomized controlled pilot trial." *J Indian Soc Pedod Prev Dent.* 2011 Apr-Jun;29(2):90–94.

Asokan S et al. "Effect of oil pulling on plaque induced gingivitis: a randomized, controlled, triple-blind study." *Indian J Dent Res.* 2009 Jan-Mar;20(1):47–51.

Asokan S et al. "Effect of oil pulling on Streptococcus mutans count in plaque and saliva using Dentocult SM Strip mutans test: a randomized, controlled, triple-blind study." *J Indian Soc Pedod Prev Dent.* 2008 Mar;26(1):12–17.

Asokan S et al. "Mechanism of oil-pulling therapy— in vitro study." *Indian J Dent Res.* 2011 Jan-Feb;22(1):33–37.

Fitzpatrick SG, Kat J. "The association between periodontal disease and cancer: A review of the literature." *Journal of Dentistry* 2010; 38:83–95.

Ide M et al. "Periodontitis and Cognitive Decline in Alzheimer's Disease." *PLOS ONE,* 2016;11 (3):e0151081. DOI: 10.1371/journal.pone.0151081.

Kaushik M et al. "The Effect of Coconut Oil pulling on Streptococcus mutans Count in Saliva in Comparison with Chlorhexidine Mouthwash." *J Contemp Dent Pract.* 2016 Jan 1;17(1):38–41.

Konig MF et al. "Aggregatibacter Actinomycetemcomitans-Induced Hypercitrullination Links Periodontal Infection to Autoimmunity in Rheumatoid Arthritis." *Sci Transl Med.* 2016 Dec 14; 8 (369), 369ra176.

Leech MT, Bartold PM. "The association between rheumatoid arthritis and periodontitis." *BPR Clin Rheum.* April 2015;29(2):189–201.

Marshall JR, Graham S, Haughey BP, et al. "Smoking, alcohol, dentition, and diet in the epidemiology of oral cancer." *Eur J Cancer B Oral Oncol* 1992; 28B:9–15.

Meyer MS, Kaumudi Joshipura, Giovannucci E, Michaud DS. "A review of the relationship between tooth loss, periodontal disease, and cancer." *Cancer Causes Control* 2008; 19:895–907.

Michaud D, Joshipura K, Giovannucci E, Fuchs C. "A prospective study of periodontal disease and pancreatic cancer in U.S. male health professionals." *J Natl Cancer Inst* 2007; 99:171–175.

Michaud DS, Liu Y, Meyer M, Giovannucci E, Joshipura K. "Periodontal disease, tooth loss, and cancer risk in male health professionals: a prospective cohort study." *Lancet Oncol* 2008; 9: 550–558.

Nishu S et al. "Effect of gum massage therapy on common pathogenic oral microorganisms—A randomized controlled trial." *J Indian Soc Periodontol.* 2014 Jul-Aug;18(4):441–446.

Peedikayil FC et al. "Effect of coconut oil in plaque related gingivitis—A preliminary report." *Niger Med J.* Mar-Apr 2015;56(2):143–147.

Smolik I, Robinson D, El-Gabalawy HS. "Periodontitis and rheumatoid arthritis: epidemiologic, clinical, and immunologic associations." *Compend Contin Educ Dent.* 2009 May;30(4):188–190,192,194.

Tezal M, Grossi SG, Genco RJ. "Is periodontitis associated with oral neoplasms?" *Journal of Periodontology* 2005; 76:406–410.

Tonetti M, D'Aiuto F, Nibali L, et al. "Treatment of periodontitis and endothelial function." *N Engl J Med* 2007; 356:911–920.

Zheng TZ, Boyle P, Hu HF, et al. "Dentition, oral hygiene, and risk of oral cancer: a case-control study in Beijing, People's Republic of China." *Cancer Causes Control* 1990; 1:235–241.

Chapter 10

Agero AL, Verallo-Rowell VM. "A randomized double-blind controlled trial comparing extra virgin coconut oil with mineral oil as a moisturizer for mild to moderate xerosis." *Dermatitis.* 2004 Sep;15(3):109–116.

Evangelista MT et al. "The effect of topical virgin coconut oil on SCORAD index, transepidermal water loss, and skin capacitance in mild to moderate pediatric atopic dermatitis: a randomized, double-blind, clinical trial." *Int J Dermatol.* 2014 Jan;53(1):100–108.

Korac RR, Khambholia KM. "Potential of herbs in skin protection from ultraviolet radiation." *Pharmacogn Rev.* 2011 Jul;5(10):164–173.

Nevin KG, T Rajamohan T. "Effect of topical application of virgin coconut oil on skin components and antioxidant status during dermal wound healing in young rats." *Skin Pharmacol Physiol.* 2010 ;23(6):290–297.

Rele AS, Mohile RB. "Effect of mineral oil, sunflower oil, and coconut oil on prevention of hair damage." *J Cosmet Sci.* Mar-Apr;54(2):175–192.

Srivastava P, Durgaprasad S. "Burn wound healing properties of Cocos nucifera: An appraisal." *Indian J Pharmacol.* 2008 Aug;40(4):144–146.

Verallo-Rowell VM et al. "Novel antibacterial and emollient effects of coconut and virgin olive oils in adult atopic dermatitis." *Dermatitis.* 2008 Nov–Dec;19(6):308–315.

Chapter 11

Samsel A and Seneff S. "Glyphosate, pathways to modern diseases II: Celiac sprue and gluten intolerance." *Interdiscip Toxicol.* 2013 Dec;6(4): 159–184.

Acknowledgments

This is another book I would not have written but for the suggestion of my friend and publisher, Rudy Shur. Thanks, Rudy.

Thanks too, to your staff at Square One who were so helpful in shepherding this book all the way to its publication, especially my editor, Erica Shur.

As always, my deepest thanks to, and appreciation for, my mother, brothers and sisters, nieces and nephews and their children, and all of my friends, without whom my life would be far less fun and love-filled.

And to my father, for the many important lessons he taught me by his example and for the way his spirit continues to guide me since his passing from this life.

About the Author

Larry Trivieri Jr is a bestselling author and nationally recognized lay authority on holistic, integrative, and non-drug-based healing methods, with more than 30 years of personal experience in exploring techniques for optimal wellness and human transformation. During that time, Trivieri has interviewed and studied with over 400 of the world's top physicians and other health practitioners in over 50 disciplines in the holistic health field.

Trivieri is the author or co-author of over 20 books on health, including *Apple Cider Vinegar: Nature's Most Versatile and Powerful Remedy*, *The Acid-Alkaline Lifestyle*, *The Acid-Alkaline Food Guide*, *Juice Alive*, *The American Holistic Medical Association Guide to Holistic Health*, *The Self-Care Guide to Holistic Medicine*, and *Health On The Edge: Visionary Views of Healing in the New Millennium*. He also served as editor and principal writer of both editions of the landmark health encyclopedia, *Alternative Medicine: The Definitive Guide*, and has written over 200 articles for Internet-based health sites. He has also written numerous feature articles for a variety of publications, including *Alternative Medicine*, for which he also served as contributing editor from 1999 through 2002; *Natural Health*, *Natural Solutions*, and *Yoga Journal*.

Trivieri is dedicated to sharing the wealth of potentially life-saving information he has learned about with as wide an audience as possible in order to help usher in a new era of wellness and health care in the 21st century. To that end, he also lectures about health nationwide, and has been a featured guest on numerous TV and radio shows across the United States.

Trivieri is also an acclaimed novelist and the author of *The Monster and Freddie Fype*, as well as the forthcoming titles *Krystle's Quest* and *Tommy's Big Question*. He lives in upstate New York.

You can follow him on Facebook at http://alturl.com/exy82 and can learn more about and purchase his other books on Amazon.com using this link: http://amzn.to/1SJFOei.

Index

Dementia, 78–80, 87-88. *See also* Alzheimer's disease.
  caused by pharmaceutical drugs, 83
  vascular, 82
Dispersal fruit, 7
Drupe, 5

Eczema, 154
Endocarp, 10
Endosperm, 10
Ephithelial tissue, 145. *See* Re-epithelialization
Essential fatty acids (EFAs), 43–44
Exocarp, 10

Fats, 33
  monosaturated, 35
  polyunsaturated, 35–26. *See* Omega fatty acids.
  saturated, 35, 46–48, 60
  trans, 36
  unsaturated, 35, 43, 60
Fiber, 32–33, 163
  coconuts as a source of, 17, 32–33
  of the coconut, 12
Framingham Heart Study, 42
Free radicals, 44, 68, 159–160, 162

Gingivitis, 140,
  study on oil pulling for treating, 145–146
Glucose, 81, 86–87
Gluten, intolerance, 164

Heart, anatomy of, 53
Heart disease, 37–38, 51
  in relation to heart disease, meta-analysis of, 58

mortality, 40. *See also* Seven Countries Study.
mortality rates, 52

High-density lipoprotein, 38
Homocysteine, 69
Hydrogenation, 36
Hyperglycemia, 81
Hypertension, 111
  essential, 112
  secondary, 113
Hypoglycemia, 81

India, 5, 7, 16
Indo-Pacific, 7
Inflammation, 37
  acute, 65
  brain, 81
  chronic, 41–45, 65–66
Kennedy, John F., 14
Ketogenic diet, 87
Ketones, 49, 86
  impact on brain function, 90-91
Ketosis, 88
Keys, Ancel 39–41. *See also* Seven Countries Study.
Kitivan study, 71–73, 117

Lauric acid, 48. *See also* Monolaurin.
LCFAs. *See* Long-chain fatty acids.
LDL cholesterol, 48. *See also* Lipoprotein(a).
Lipoprotein(a), 68
Long-chain fatty acids (LCFAs), 48–50, 129–131
Lou Gehrig's disease (ALS), 90, 94
Low-density lipoprotein (LDL), 38, 42, 49, 68. *See also* Oxidized cholesterol.

Other Square One Titles of Interest

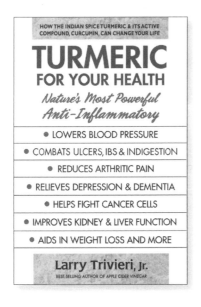

Turmeric for Your Health

Nature's Most Powerful Anti-Inflammatory

Larry Trivieri, Jr.

Imagine a natural spice that has the power to reduce or eliminate inflammation, the underlying cause of many serious health disorders. For over 5,000 years, India's Ayurvedic medical practitioners have used turmeric to treat a host of painful and debilitating diseases. Recently, medical researchers in the US have turned their attention to this ancient root and have discovered its effectiveness in lowering blood pressure, reducing arthritis pain, combating gastrointestinal issues, increasing brain function, aiding in weight loss, and much more. *Turmeric for Your Health* is a simple guide to understanding the science behind turmeric's effectiveness. Along with breakthrough research, it presents an A-to-Z listing of ailments for which turmeric can provide successful treatment. With few if any side effects, turmeric can offer a safe, inexpensive way to enhance your health and well-being.

March • $15.95 US • 192 pages •
6 x 9-inch paperback • ISBN 978-0-7570-0452-0

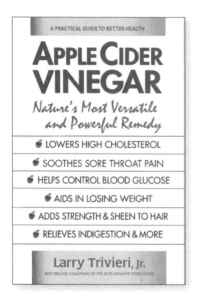

A PRACTICAL GUIDE TO BETTER HEALTH

APPLE CIDER VINEGAR

Nature's Most Versatile and Powerful Remedy

✔ LOWERS HIGH CHOLESTEROL

✔ SOOTHES SORE THROAT PAIN

✔ HELPS CONTROL BLOOD GLUCOSE

✔ AIDS IN LOSING WEIGHT

✔ ADDS STRENGTH & SHEEN TO HAIR

✔ RELIEVES INDIGESTION & MORE

Larry Trivieri, Jr.

BEST-SELLING COAUTHOR OF THE ACID ALKALINE FOOD GUIDE

Apple Cider Vinegar

Nature's Most Versatile and Powerful Remedy

Larry Trivieri, Jr.

For centuries, apple cider vinegar has been used as a folk remedy to treat a host of health issues, from indigestion and low energy to sore throats and toothache. It is also a remarkable beauty aid that can help remove unwanted blemishes and add strength and sheen to hair. And that's just the tip of what this amazing elixir can do.

Best-selling health author Larry Trivieri, Jr. has written this practical guide to the many well-known benefits of apple cider as well as the elixir's newly discovered powers as a natural anti-inflammatory.

This book begins by looking at the long history of apple cider vinegar use and examines the science behind its many benefits. It then explains how you can choose the best apple cider vinegar, and even tells you how to make it at home. The main section of this book is a complete A-Z guide that shows you how to use apple cider vinegar to prevent and reverse over 80 common health conditions, and to improve and maintain the health and appearance of your hair, skin, teeth and gums. Each entry includes a clear discussion of the topic, explains how and why apple cider vinegar works to help each condition, and then guides you on how to most effectively use it.

Apple Cider Vinegar is the most complete and comprehensive book of its kind. By applying what you will learn in it, you will take an important step to better and longer lasting health.

$14.95 US • 240 pages • 6 x 9-inch paperback • ISBN 978-0-7570-0446-9